10 Superfoods

A Practical Guide to Transform Your Health
with Nature's Best Nutrient-Rich Foods

Conard Howe

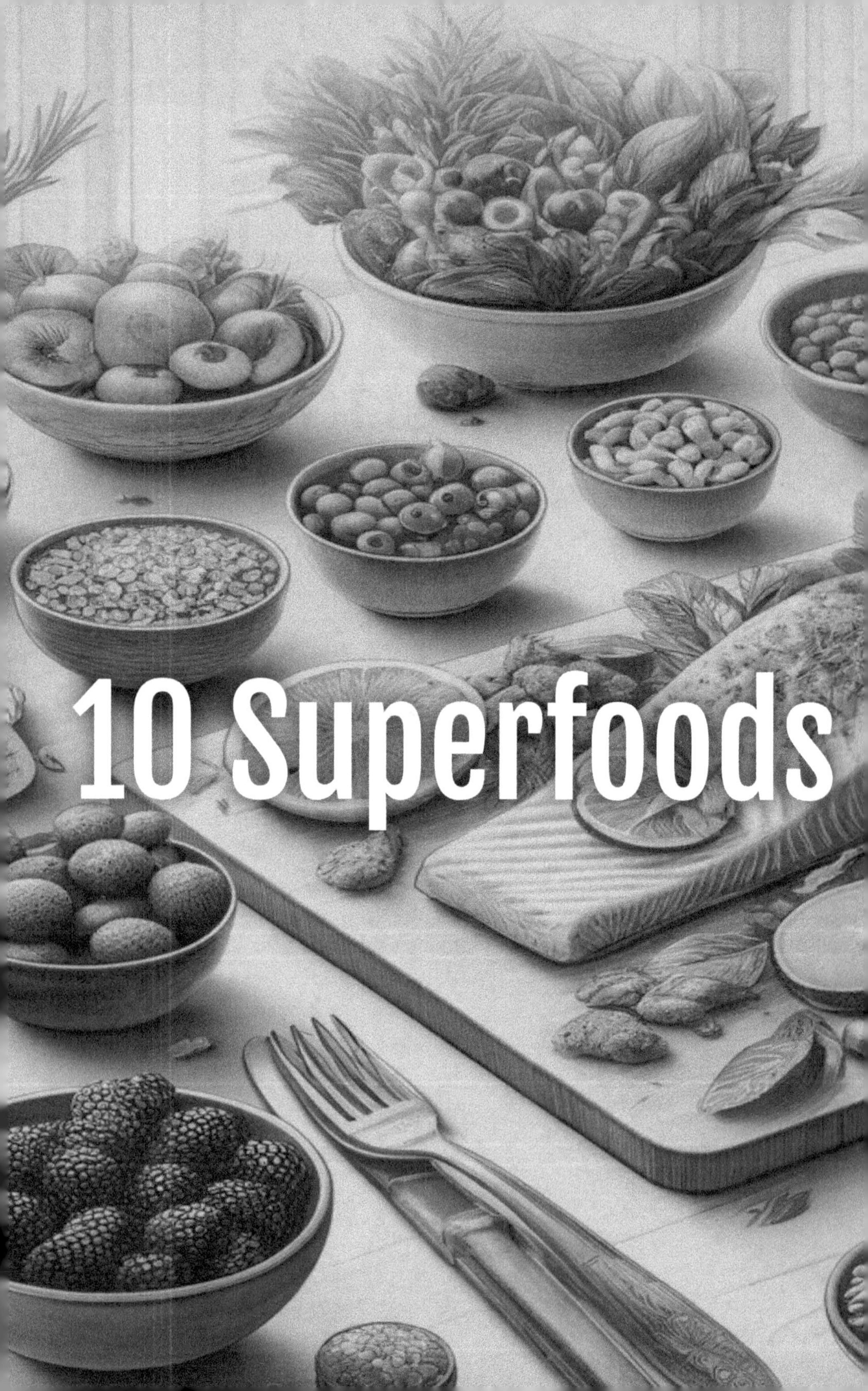

10 Superfoods

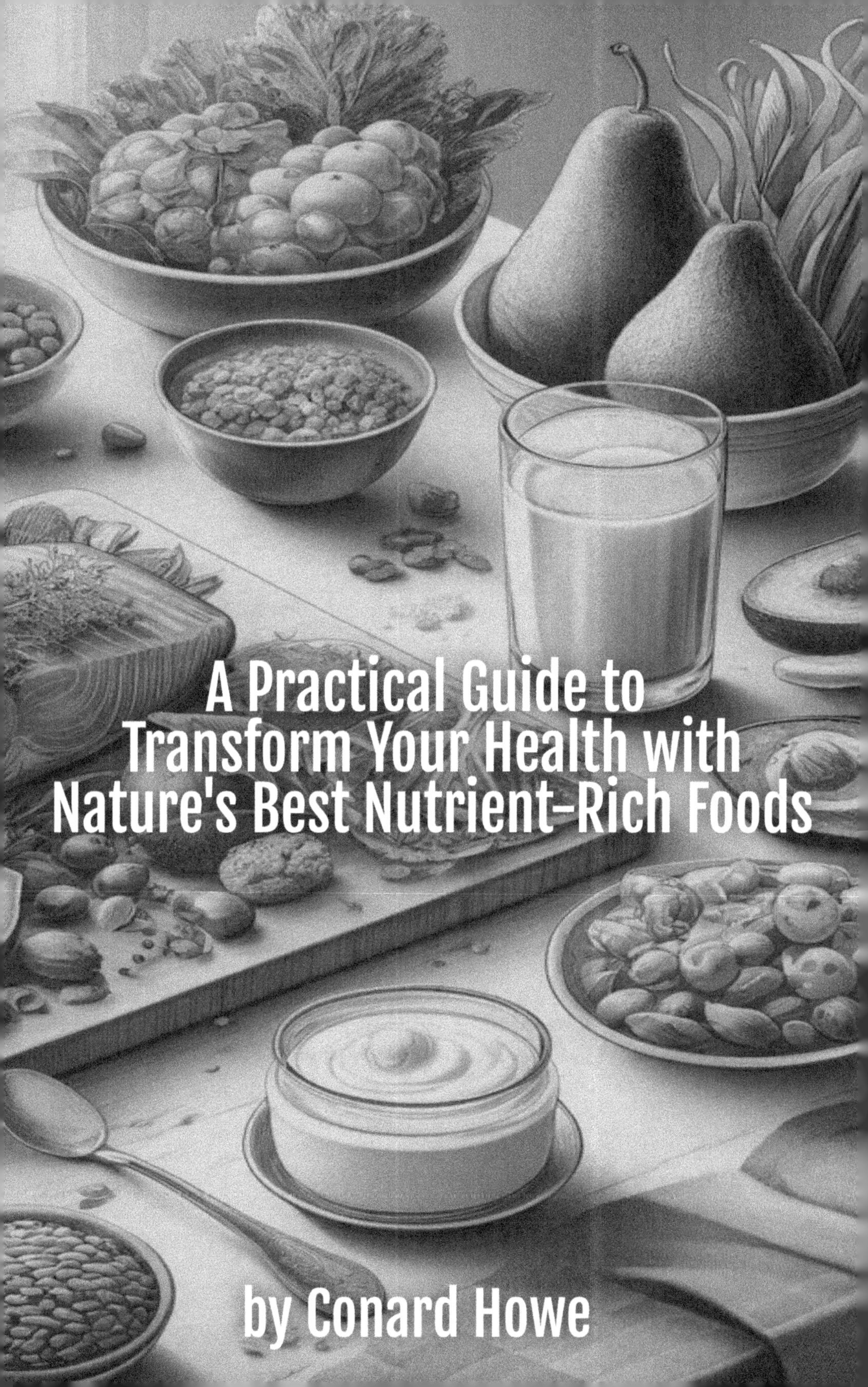

A Practical Guide to Transform Your Health with Nature's Best Nutrient-Rich Foods
by Conard Howe

Contents

Introduction

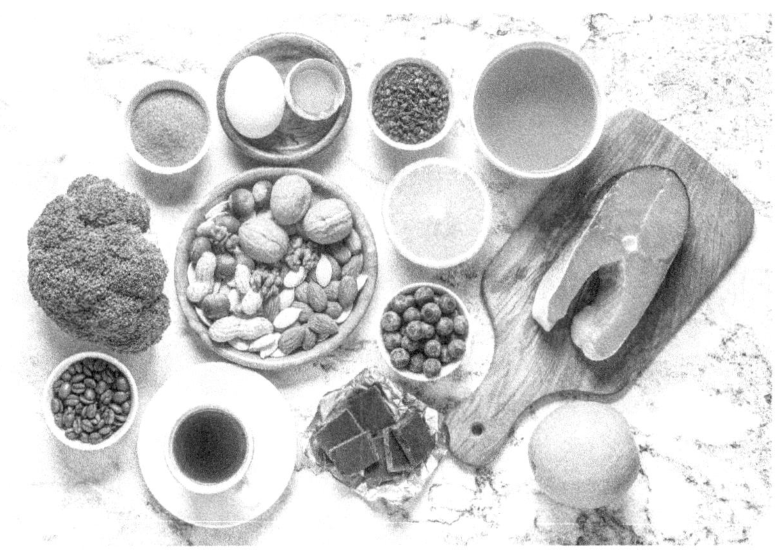

Welcome to a journey into the world of superfoods, where we delve into the incredible power of nutrition to transform your health and well-being. Superfoods are not just a trendy buzzword; they are nutrient-rich foods that provide an abundance of essential vitamins, minerals, and antioxidants that your body needs to function at its best. These foods can be fruits, vegetables, grains, or even herbs, each offering unique health benefits that can significantly impact your life.

The purpose of this book is to educate and inspire you to incorporate these superfoods into your daily diet. I have carefully selected ten superfoods that are not only packed with nutrition but also versatile and delicious. From common staples like spinach and blueberries to exciting finds like chia seeds and quinoa, we will explore how each of these foods can contribute to your overall health.

My goal in writing this book is to provide you with the knowledge and tools needed to make informed choices about what you eat. I believe that by understanding the specific benefits of these superfoods, you can take proactive steps towards improving your health. Whether you want to boost your immune system, support your heart health, improve your digestive system, or simply increase your energy levels, this book has something for you.

As you read through each chapter, you will discover detailed information about the nutritional profiles of these superfoods, the science behind their health benefits, and practical tips on how to incorporate them into your meals. Additionally, I have included a variety of recipes to help you enjoy these superfoods in delicious and creative ways.

By the end of this book, you will not only have a deeper understanding of what superfoods are and why they are beneficial, but you will also be equipped with actionable strategies to integrate them into your daily routine. My hope is to inspire you to make small, manageable changes that can lead to significant improvements in your health.

So lets do it! Get ready because your journey to better health starts now. Together, we will unlock the power of superfoods and help you achieve a healthier, more vibrant life.

Kale

The Nutrient-Dense Powerhouse

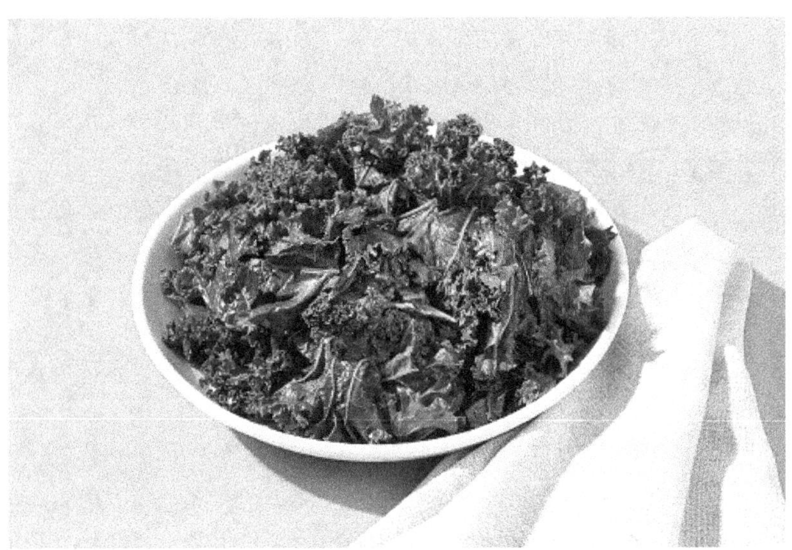

Welcome to the leafy green giant of the vegetable world: kale. Often heralded as a superfood, kale is more than just a health trend. Its rich nutrient profile and versatility make it an invaluable addition to any diet. This chapter will explore kale's nutritional benefits, delve into its specific contributions to our health, and provide practical tips and recipes to help you incorporate this powerhouse green into your daily meals.

The Nutritional Profile of Kale

Kale stands out for its remarkable nutritional richness. A single cup of raw kale contains:

- Vitamin A: 206% of the Daily Value (DV)

- Vitamin C: 134% of the DV

- Vitamin K: 684% of the DV

- Calcium: 9% of the DV

- Potassium: 6% of the DV

- Fiber: 2 grams

This combination of vitamins and minerals makes kale a standout in the world of leafy greens. Its high vitamin K content is particularly notable, as few foods offer such a concentrated source of this crucial nutrient.

Kale's Role in Bone Health

One of the standout benefits of kale is its ability to support and enhance bone health. Here's how it works:

The Power of Vitamin K

Vitamin K is essential for bone health because it helps in the regulation of calcium absorption and bone mineralization. When you consume adequate amounts of vitamin K, you enable your body to deposit calcium into your bones effectively, thereby improving bone density and reducing the risk of fractures and osteoporosis. Studies have shown that a diet high in vitamin K can improve bone health outcomes, especially in postmenopausal women who are at increased risk of osteoporosis.

Calcium Content

While kale might not be the first food you think of when it comes to calcium, it's an excellent plant-based source. A cup of cooked kale provides a substantial amount of calcium, which is vital for maintaining bone structure and function. For those who are lactose intolerant or prefer not to consume dairy, kale offers an alternative way to ensure you're meeting your calcium needs.

Boosting Immunity with Kale

Kale's impressive vitamin C content makes it a powerful ally for your immune system. Here's how:

Antioxidant Protection

Vitamin C is a potent antioxidant that protects your cells from damage by free radicals. By neutralizing these harmful molecules, vitamin C helps reduce inflammation and supports the immune system in fighting off infections.

Enhancing Immune Function

Vitamin C is also crucial for the production and function of white blood cells, which are the body's primary defense against infection. Consuming kale regularly can help ensure that your immune system remains robust and ready to tackle any pathogens it encounters.

Promoting Healthy Skin with Kale

Kale contributes to skin health in several ways, primarily through its high levels of vitamins A and C.

Collagen Production

Vitamin C plays a key role in collagen synthesis, a process that keeps your skin firm and elastic. Collagen is a protein that provides structure to your skin, and adequate vitamin C intake is necessary for the body to produce this vital protein. By consuming kale, you support your skin's ability to repair itself and maintain its youthful appearance.

UV Protection

Vitamin A in kale helps protect your skin from UV damage. While it's not a substitute for sunscreen, vitamin A can enhance your skin's resilience to the harmful effects of sun exposure.

Skin Cell Turnover

Both vitamins A and C contribute to skin cell turnover, a process that keeps your skin looking fresh and vibrant. By regularly including kale in your diet, you can help reduce the appearance of wrinkles and maintain a glowing complexion.

Delicious Ways to Enjoy Kale

Incorporating kale into your diet doesn't have to be a chore. Here are some tasty and easy ways to enjoy this superfood:

Raw Kale Salads

Raw kale can be tough and bitter, but with the right preparation, it can be delicious. Massage kale leaves with a bit of olive oil and lemon juice until they become tender. This simple technique breaks down the fibrous texture and enhances the flavor. Add your favorite salad toppings such as avocado, nuts, seeds, and a tangy dressing for a nutritious and satisfying meal.

Kale in Soups and Stews

Adding kale to soups and stews is a great way to boost the nutritional content of these dishes. Simply chop the leaves and stir them in during the last few minutes of cooking. Kale's sturdy texture holds up well to heat, making it a perfect addition to hearty soups and stews.

Smoothies and Juices

Blend kale into smoothies or juices for an easy way to consume more greens. Pair it with fruits like bananas, apples, and berries to balance the earthy flavor. A handful of kale in your morning smoothie can set you up for a day of healthy eating.

Kale Chips

For a healthy snack, try making kale chips. Toss kale leaves with a bit of olive oil and your favorite seasonings, then bake them in a single layer at a low temperature until crispy. Kale chips are a satisfying and nutritious alternative to traditional potato chips.

Kale Recipes to Try

Here are a few delicious recipes to help you get started with incorporating more kale into your diet:

Massaged Kale Salad with Avocado and Nuts

Ingredients:

- 1 bunch of kale, stems removed and leaves chopped

- 1 avocado, diced

- 1/4 cup of nuts (almonds, walnuts, or pecans)

- 1/4 cup of dried cranberries

- Juice of 1 lemon

- 2 tablespoons of olive oil

- Salt and pepper to taste

Instructions:

1. Place the chopped kale in a large bowl.

2. Drizzle with olive oil and lemon juice.

3. Massage the kale with your hands for a few minutes until it becomes tender.

4. Add the diced avocado, nuts, and dried cranberries.

5. Season with salt and pepper, then toss to combine.

6. Serve immediately and enjoy.

Hearty Kale and White Bean Soup

Ingredients:

- 1 tablespoon of olive oil

- 1 onion, chopped

- 2 cloves of garlic, minced

- 1 carrot, diced

- 1 celery stalk, diced

- 1 can of white beans, drained and rinsed

- 4 cups of vegetable broth

- 1 bunch of kale, stems removed and leaves chopped

- Salt and pepper to taste

Instructions:

1. Heat the olive oil in a large pot over medium heat.

2. Add the onion, garlic, carrot, and celery, and sauté until the vegetables are soft.

3. Stir in the white beans and vegetable broth.

4. Bring to a boil, then reduce heat and simmer for 10 minutes.

5. Add the kale and cook until wilted, about 5 minutes.

6. Season with salt and pepper to taste.

7. Serve hot with a slice of crusty bread.

Kale and Berry Smoothie

Ingredients:

- 1 cup of kale leaves, packed

- 1 banana

- 1/2 cup of frozen berries (blueberries, strawberries, or raspberries)

- 1 cup of almond milk or any milk of your choice

- 1 tablespoon of chia seeds

- 1 teaspoon of honey (optional)

Instructions:

1. Place all ingredients in a blender.

2. Blend until smooth.

3. Pour into a glass and enjoy immediately.

Baked Kale Chips

Ingredients:

- 1 bunch of kale, stems removed and leaves torn into bite-sized pieces

- 1 tablespoon of olive oil

- Salt to taste

- Optional seasonings: garlic powder, paprika, nutritional yeast

Instructions:

1. Preheat your oven to 300°F (150°C).

2. In a large bowl, toss the kale pieces with olive oil until evenly coated.

3. Spread the kale in a single layer on a baking sheet.

4. Sprinkle with salt and any optional seasonings.

5. Bake for 20-25 minutes, or until the kale is crispy, but not burnt.

6. Allow to cool before serving.

Kale's incredible nutritional profile makes it a standout superfood that can significantly benefit your health. From supporting bone health and boosting immunity to promoting healthy skin, the advantages of including kale in your diet are numerous. With the practical tips and delicious recipes provided, you can easily make kale a regular part of your meals and enjoy its many benefits. This nutrient-dense leafy green can transform your overall health one delicious bite at a time.

Chapter Two

Blueberries

The Antioxidant-Rich Powerhouses

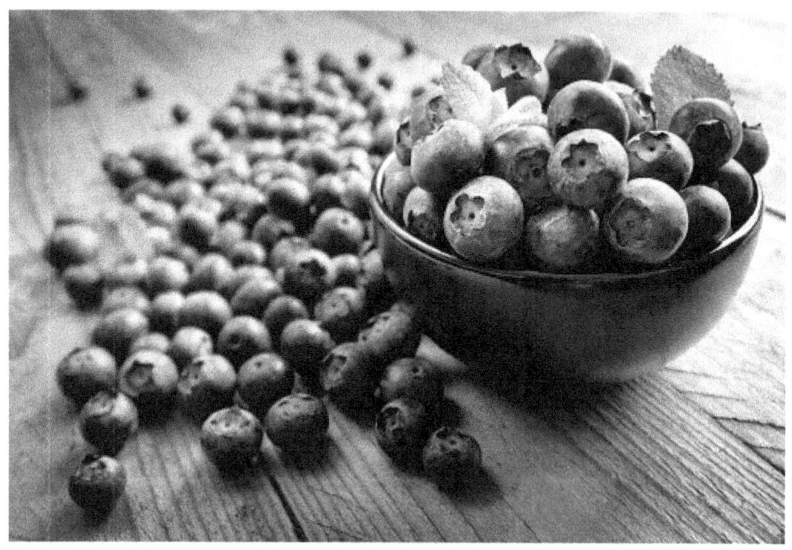

B lueberries, often referred to as nature's candy, are more than just a delicious treat. These small, vibrant berries are packed with powerful antioxidants that offer a myriad of health benefits. In this chapter, we'll explore the nutritional profile of blueberries, their specific health benefits, and provide practical tips and recipes to help you incorporate these super berries into your daily diet.

The Nutritional Profile of Blueberries

Blueberries are low in calories but high in nutrients. A one-cup serving (about 148 grams) of blueberries contains:

- Calories: 84

- Fiber: 4 grams

- Vitamin C: 24% of the Daily Value (DV)

- Vitamin K: 36% of the DV

- Manganese: 25% of the DV

Blueberries are also a rich source of anthocyanins, the antioxidants that give them their deep blue color. These compounds play a key role in the numerous health benefits attributed to blueberries.

Blueberries and Cognitive Function

One of the most compelling reasons to include blueberries in your diet is their potential to enhance cognitive function. Here's how blueberries benefit brain health:

Protection Against Oxidative Stress

Blueberries are high in antioxidants, particularly anthocyanins, which help protect brain cells from oxidative stress. Oxidative stress can lead to inflammation and damage to brain cells, contributing to cognitive decline and neurodegenerative diseases. Regular consumption of blueberries can help mitigate these effects, preserving brain health as you age.

Improved Memory and Cognitive Function

Studies have shown that the antioxidants in blueberries can improve memory and cognitive function. In older adults, regular consumption of blueberries has been linked to better memory performance and delayed cognitive aging. These benefits are thought to result from the anti-inflammatory and neuroprotective effects of the compounds found in blueberries.

Blueberries and Heart Health

Blueberries are also known for their heart-protective properties. Here's how they support cardiovascular health:

Reducing Oxidative Stress and Inflammation

The antioxidants in blueberries help reduce oxidative stress and inflammation, two major contributors to heart disease. By neutralizing free radicals, blueberries can help prevent the damage that leads to the buildup of plaque in the arteries, reducing the risk of heart attacks and strokes.

Improving Cholesterol Levels

Regular consumption of blueberries has been associated with improved cholesterol profiles. The antioxidants in blueberries can help increase levels of HDL (good) cholesterol and reduce levels of LDL (bad) cholesterol, which is essential for maintaining a healthy heart.

Lowering Blood Pressure

Anthocyanins, the compounds that give blueberries their color, have been shown to help lower blood pressure. Some studies suggest that eating blueberries regularly can lead to significant reductions in both systolic and diastolic blood pressure. This effect is particularly beneficial for individuals with hypertension, a major risk factor for heart disease.

How to Enjoy Blueberries

Incorporating blueberries into your diet is easy and enjoyable. Here are some delicious ways to add these antioxidant-rich berries to your meals:

Fresh Blueberries as a Snack

One of the simplest ways to enjoy blueberries is to eat them fresh. They make a perfect snack on their own or can be mixed into yogurt, oatmeal, or cereal for a burst of flavor and nutrition. The natural sweetness of blueberries pairs well with a variety of foods, making them a versatile addition to any meal.

Blueberry Smoothies

Frozen blueberries are an excellent ingredient for smoothies. They add a natural sweetness and vibrant color while boosting the nutritional content. Blend blueberries with other fruits, vegetables, and a liquid base like almond milk or coconut water for a refreshing and healthy beverage.

Baking with Blueberries

Blueberries can be added to pancakes, muffins, and other baked goods for a delicious and nutritious boost. Their sweet-tart flavor enhances a variety of recipes, making them a favorite in the kitchen.

Try incorporating blueberries into your favorite baking recipes for an added health benefit.

Blueberries in Salads and Sauces

For a unique twist, try adding blueberries to salads or using them in sauces. Their sweet and tangy flavor complements savory dishes beautifully. A handful of blueberries can brighten up a green salad, or you can cook them down into a sauce to serve with meats or desserts.

Blueberry Recipes to Try

Here are a few delicious recipes to help you get started with incorporating more blueberries into your diet:

Blueberry and Greek Yogurt Parfait

Ingredients:

- 1 cup of fresh blueberries

- 1 cup of Greek yogurt

- 1 tablespoon of honey

- 1/4 cup of granola

- Mint leaves for garnish

Instructions:

1. In a glass or bowl, layer half of the Greek yogurt.

2. Add half of the blueberries and drizzle with honey.

3. Repeat the layers with the remaining yogurt and blueberries.

4. Top with granola and garnish with mint leaves.

5. Serve immediately and enjoy.

Blueberry Spinach Salad

Ingredients:

- 2 cups of fresh spinach leaves

- 1 cup of fresh blueberries

- 1/4 cup of crumbled feta cheese

- 1/4 cup of sliced almonds

- 1/4 red onion, thinly sliced

- 2 tablespoons of balsamic vinaigrette

Instructions:

1. In a large bowl, combine the spinach, blueberries, feta

cheese, sliced almonds, and red onion.

2. Drizzle with balsamic vinaigrette and toss to combine.

3. Serve immediately as a refreshing and nutritious salad.

Blueberry Smoothie

Ingredients:

- 1 cup of frozen blueberries

- 1 banana

- 1/2 cup of Greek yogurt

- 1 cup of almond milk

- 1 tablespoon of honey (optional)

- 1 teaspoon of chia seeds (optional)

Instructions:

1. Place all ingredients in a blender.

2. Blend until smooth.

3. Pour into a glass and enjoy immediately.

Blueberry Muffins

Ingredients:

- 1 1/2 cups of all-purpose flour

- 1/2 cup of sugar

- 1/2 teaspoon of salt

- 2 teaspoons of baking powder

- 1/3 cup of vegetable oil

- 1 egg

- 1/3 cup of milk

- 1 cup of fresh blueberries

Instructions:

1. Preheat your oven to 400°F (200°C). Grease a muffin tin or line with muffin cups.

2. In a medium bowl, mix together the flour, sugar, salt, and baking powder.

3. In a separate bowl, combine the vegetable oil, egg, and milk.

4. Stir the wet ingredients into the dry ingredients until just

combined.

5. Fold in the blueberries gently.

6. Fill the muffin cups about 2/3 full.

7. Bake for 20-25 minutes, or until a toothpick inserted into the center comes out clean.

8. Allow to cool before serving.

Blueberries are a true superfood, packed with antioxidants that provide numerous health benefits. From improving cognitive function and protecting against heart disease to helping lower blood pressure, the advantages of adding blueberries to your diet are undeniable. With the practical tips and delicious recipes provided, you can easily make blueberries a regular part of your meals and enjoy their many benefits. These antioxidant-rich berries can transform your health one delicious bite at a time.

Chapter Three

Salmon

- -

The Omega-3 Powerhouse

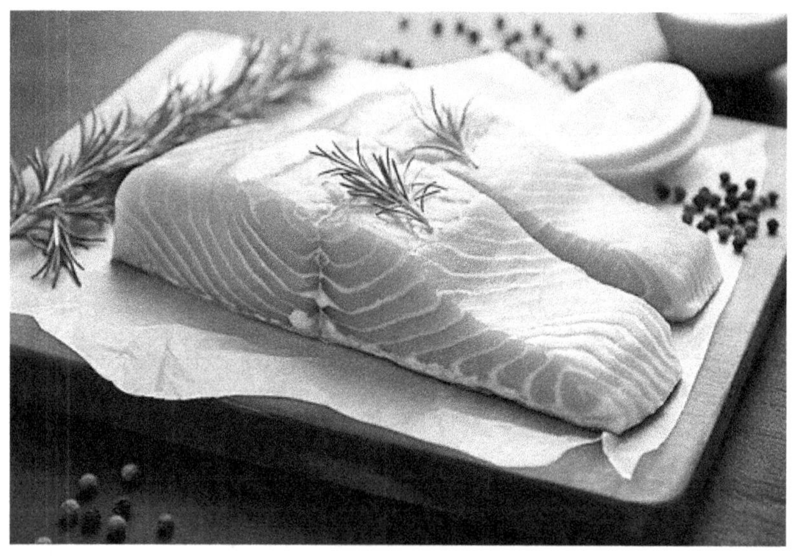

Salmon, renowned for its rich, savory flavor and versatile culinary uses, is also a nutritional powerhouse. This chapter delves into the numerous health benefits of salmon, focusing on its high content of omega-3 fatty acids, particularly EPA (eicosapentaenoic acid) and

DHA (docosahexaenoic acid). We will explore the specific health benefits of these essential fats, practical tips for incorporating salmon into your diet, and provide delicious recipes to make the most of this remarkable fish.

The Nutritional Profile of Salmon

Salmon is packed with essential nutrients that contribute to overall health. A 3.5-ounce (100-gram) serving of wild-caught salmon contains:

- Calories: 206

- Protein: 22 grams

- Fat: 12 grams (including 2 grams of omega-3 fatty acids)

- Vitamin D: 82% of the Daily Value (DV)

- Vitamin B12: 117% of the DV

- Selenium: 52% of the DV

The Omega-3 Benefits of Salmon

Salmon's high content of omega-3 fatty acids, particularly EPA and DHA, is responsible for many of its health benefits. Here's how these essential fats enhance your health:

Supporting Heart Health

Omega-3 fatty acids are crucial for heart health. They help reduce inflammation, lower triglyceride levels, and improve blood vessel function, all of which contribute to a healthier cardiovascular system. Here's a closer look:

Reducing Inflammation

Inflammation is a natural response to injury or infection, but chronic inflammation can lead to various health problems, including heart disease. Omega-3 fatty acids have potent anti-inflammatory properties, helping to reduce inflammation throughout the body. By consuming salmon regularly, you can lower inflammation markers and support overall heart health.

Lowering Triglycerides

High levels of triglycerides in the blood are a risk factor for heart disease. Omega-3 fatty acids in salmon have been shown to lower triglyceride levels, thereby reducing the risk of cardiovascular issues. Regular consumption of salmon can help maintain healthy triglyceride levels and promote better heart health.

Improving Blood Vessel Function

Omega-3s also improve the function of blood vessels by enhancing endothelial function (the lining of the blood vessels). This can lead to better blood flow and reduced blood pressure. By incorporating salmon into your diet, you can support healthy blood vessel function and reduce the risk of heart disease and stroke.

Reducing Inflammation with Salmon

Chronic inflammation is linked to a range of health issues, including arthritis, heart disease, and certain cancers. The anti-inflammatory properties of the omega-3 fatty acids in salmon can help mitigate these risks.

Arthritis Relief

For individuals suffering from arthritis, omega-3 fatty acids can provide relief by reducing joint pain and stiffness. Studies have shown that regular consumption of omega-3-rich foods like salmon can improve symptoms of rheumatoid arthritis and other inflammatory joint conditions.

Cancer Prevention

While research is ongoing, some studies suggest that omega-3 fatty acids may help reduce the risk of certain cancers by reducing inflammation and inhibiting the growth of cancer cells. Including salmon in your diet as part of a balanced, anti-inflammatory eating plan can support overall health and potentially lower cancer risk.

Promoting Brain Function with Salmon

DHA, a type of omega-3 fatty acid found in salmon, is crucial for brain health and cognitive function. Here's how it supports your brain:

Brain Structure and Function

DHA is an essential component of brain cell membranes, playing a critical role in maintaining the structure and function of brain cells. Adequate DHA levels are necessary for optimal brain function, supporting processes such as memory, learning, and mood regulation.

Cognitive Decline Prevention

Regular consumption of DHA-rich foods like salmon has been linked to a reduced risk of age-related cognitive decline and neurodegenerative diseases. Studies have shown that individuals who consume more omega-3s have a lower risk of Alzheimer's disease and other forms of dementia.

Mood Regulation

Omega-3 fatty acids also play a role in mood regulation and mental health. Some studies suggest that omega-3s can help reduce symptoms of depression and anxiety. Including salmon in your diet may support better mental health and overall well-being.

Delicious Ways to Enjoy Salmon

Incorporating salmon into your diet can be both easy and delicious. Here are some flavorful ways to enjoy this omega-3-rich fish:

Grilled or Baked Salmon

Grilling or baking salmon fillets is a simple and healthy way to prepare this fish. Here's a basic recipe:

Ingredients:

- 4 salmon fillets

- 2 tablespoons of olive oil

- Juice of 1 lemon

- 2 garlic cloves, minced

- 1 teaspoon of dried dill

- Salt and pepper to taste

Instructions:

1. Preheat your grill or oven to 400°F (200°C).

2. In a small bowl, combine olive oil, lemon juice, garlic, dill, salt, and pepper.

3. Brush the salmon fillets with the mixture.

4. Grill or bake for 12-15 minutes, or until the salmon is cooked through and flakes easily with a fork.

5. Serve with a side of vegetables or a salad.

Flaked Salmon in Salads and Pasta

Adding flaked salmon to salads and pasta dishes is an easy way to boost protein and omega-3 intake. Here's a simple pasta recipe:

Ingredients:

- 8 ounces of whole-grain pasta

- 2 salmon fillets, cooked and flaked

- 2 cups of cherry tomatoes, halved

- 1/4 cup of fresh basil, chopped

- 2 tablespoons of olive oil

- Juice of 1 lemon

- Salt and pepper to taste

Instructions:

1. Cook the pasta according to package instructions.

2. In a large bowl, combine the cooked pasta, flaked salmon, cherry tomatoes, and basil.

3. Drizzle with olive oil and lemon juice.

4. Season with salt and pepper, then toss to combine.

5. Serve warm or cold.

Salmon Burgers or Patties

Salmon burgers or patties are a delicious and versatile option. Here's a basic recipe using canned salmon:

Ingredients:

- 1 can of salmon, drained and flaked

- 1/4 cup of breadcrumbs

- 1 egg, beaten

- 2 tablespoons of fresh parsley, chopped

- 1 garlic clove, minced

- Salt and pepper to taste

- Olive oil for cooking

Instructions:

1. In a large bowl, combine the flaked salmon, breadcrumbs, egg, parsley, garlic, salt, and pepper.

2. Form the mixture into patties.

3. Heat olive oil in a skillet over medium heat.

4. Cook the patties for 3-4 minutes on each side, or until golden brown and cooked through.

5. Serve on whole-grain buns with your favorite toppings.

Salmon Recipes to Try

Here are a few more delicious recipes to help you incorporate salmon into your diet:

Lemon Herb Baked Salmon

Ingredients:

- 4 salmon fillets

- 2 tablespoons of olive oil

- Juice of 1 lemon

- 1 teaspoon of dried thyme

- 1 teaspoon of dried rosemary

- Salt and pepper to taste

Instructions:

1. Preheat your oven to 400°F (200°C).

2. In a small bowl, combine olive oil, lemon juice, thyme, rosemary, salt, and pepper.

3. Brush the salmon fillets with the mixture.

4. Place the salmon fillets on a baking sheet lined with parchment paper.

5. Bake for 12-15 minutes, or until the salmon is cooked through and flakes easily with a fork.

6. Serve with steamed vegetables or a fresh salad.

Teriyaki Salmon

Ingredients:

- 4 salmon fillets

- 1/4 cup of soy sauce

- 2 tablespoons of honey

- 1 tablespoon of rice vinegar

- 2 garlic cloves, minced

- 1 teaspoon of grated ginger

- Sesame seeds and green onions for garnish

Instructions:

1. In a small bowl, combine soy sauce, honey, rice vinegar, garlic, and ginger.

2. Place the salmon fillets in a shallow dish and pour the marinade over them. Let marinate for at least 30 minutes.

3. Preheat your grill or oven to 400°F (200°C).

4. Grill or bake the salmon for 12-15 minutes, or until cooked through.

5. Garnish with sesame seeds and green onions before serving.

Salmon and Avocado Salad

Ingredients:

- 2 salmon fillets, cooked and flaked

- 1 avocado, diced

- 4 cups of mixed greens

- 1/2 cup of cherry tomatoes, halved

- 1/4 cup of red onion, thinly sliced

- 2 tablespoons of olive oil

- Juice of 1 lime

- Salt and pepper to taste

Instructions:

1. In a large bowl, combine the mixed greens, flaked salmon, avocado, cherry tomatoes, and red onion.

2. Drizzle with olive oil and lime juice.

3. Season with salt and pepper, then toss to combine.

4. Serve immediately as a refreshing and nutritious salad.

Salmon is an exceptional source of omega-3 fatty acids, providing numerous health benefits including supporting heart health, reducing inflammation, and promoting brain function. By incorporating salmon into your diet through the practical tips and delicious recipes provided, you can enjoy the many advantages of this nutrient-rich fish. The omega-3 powerhouse that is salmon can transform your health one delectable meal at a time.

Chapter Four

Spinach

The Nutrient-Rich Leafy Green

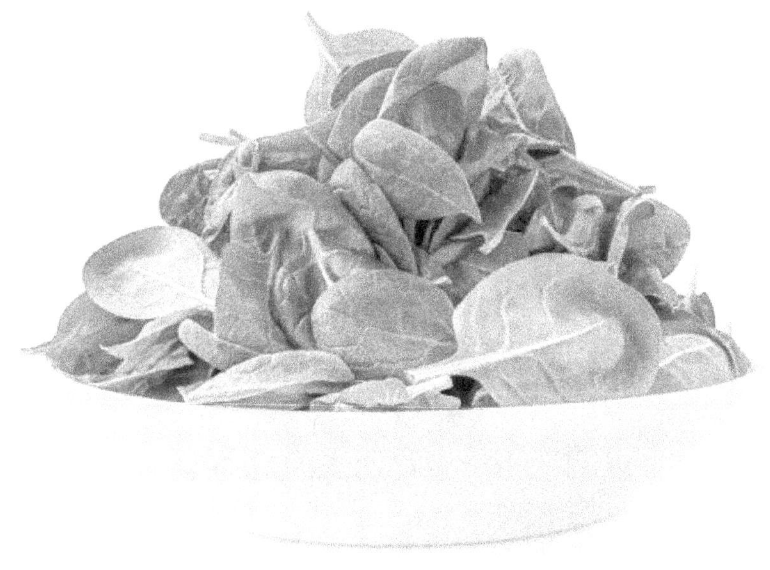

Spinach, a beloved leafy green, is celebrated for its rich nutrient profile and versatility in the kitchen. From boosting bone health to supporting digestion and enhancing eyesight, spinach offers a wide range of health benefits. In this chapter, we'll delve into the nutritional content of spinach, explore its specific health benefits, and provide practical tips and recipes to help you incorporate this superfood into your daily meals.

The Nutritional Profile of Spinach

Spinach is incredibly nutrient-dense, providing a host of essential vitamins and minerals in a low-calorie package. A 100-gram serving of raw spinach contains:

- Calories: 23

- Protein: 2.9 grams

- Carbohydrates: 3.6 grams

- Fiber: 2.2 grams

- Vitamin A: 188% of the Daily Value (DV)

- Vitamin C: 47% of the DV

- Vitamin K: 604% of the DV

- Iron: 21% of the DV

- Folate: 49% of the DV

In addition to these nutrients, spinach is rich in antioxidants, including lutein and zeaxanthin, which play crucial roles in maintaining overall health.

Spinach and Bone Health

Spinach is a powerhouse for bone health, thanks to its high vitamin K content. Here's how it supports strong bones:

The Role of Vitamin K

Vitamin K is essential for bone health because it helps the body use calcium to build and maintain bones. It activates proteins that are involved in bone formation and mineralization. Adequate vitamin K intake is associated with higher bone density and a reduced risk of fractures.

Calcium Content

Although not as high in calcium as dairy products, spinach still provides a significant amount of this important mineral. Combined with its vitamin K content, spinach helps support a healthy skeletal system.

Aiding Digestion with Spinach

Spinach is a digestive superhero, largely due to its fiber content. Here's how it promotes digestive health:

Fiber for Digestive Health

Fiber is essential for a healthy digestive system. It adds bulk to the stool and helps it move smoothly through the digestive tract, preventing constipation. A diet high in fiber can promote regular bowel movements and prevent digestive issues like irritable bowel syndrome (IBS).

Promoting Gut Health

The fiber in spinach also acts as a prebiotic, feeding the beneficial bacteria in your gut. A healthy gut microbiome is crucial for overall health, including improved digestion, enhanced immune function, and reduced inflammation.

Supporting Healthy Eyesight

Spinach is packed with nutrients that are essential for maintaining good vision. Here's how it helps protect your eyesight:

Vitamin A

Vitamin A is vital for eye health, and spinach is an excellent source of this nutrient. It helps maintain the health of the cornea and supports night vision. A deficiency in vitamin A can lead to vision problems, including night blindness.

Lutein and Zeaxanthin

Spinach is rich in antioxidants like lutein and zeaxanthin, which are concentrated in the retina and help protect the eyes from damage caused by blue light and UV rays. These antioxidants can reduce the risk of age-related macular degeneration (AMD) and cataracts, keeping your vision sharp as you age.

Delicious Ways to Enjoy Spinach

Incorporating spinach into your diet can be both easy and delicious. Here are some tasty ways to add this nutrient-rich green to your meals:

Spinach in Salads and Wraps

Fresh spinach makes a fantastic base for salads and can be added to wraps for an extra boost of nutrients. Here's a simple salad recipe:

Ingredients:

- 4 cups of fresh spinach leaves

- 1/2 cup of cherry tomatoes, halved

- 1/4 cup of red onion, thinly sliced

- 1/4 cup of feta cheese, crumbled

- 2 tablespoons of olive oil

- 1 tablespoon of balsamic vinegar

- Salt and pepper to taste

Instructions:

1. In a large bowl, combine the spinach, cherry tomatoes, red onion, and feta cheese.

2. Drizzle with olive oil and balsamic vinegar.

3. Season with salt and pepper, then toss to combine.

4. Serve immediately.

Spinach in Soups and Stews

Adding spinach to soups and stews is an easy way to boost their nutritional content. Here's a hearty soup recipe:

Ingredients:

- 1 tablespoon of olive oil

- 1 onion, chopped

- 2 garlic cloves, minced

- 2 carrots, sliced

- 2 celery stalks, sliced

- 4 cups of vegetable broth

- 1 can of white beans, drained and rinsed

- 4 cups of fresh spinach leaves

- Salt and pepper to taste

Instructions:

1. Heat the olive oil in a large pot over medium heat.

2. Add the onion, garlic, carrots, and celery, and sauté until the vegetables are tender.

3. Stir in the vegetable broth and white beans.

4. Bring to a boil, then reduce heat and simmer for 10 minutes.

5. Add the spinach and cook until wilted, about 2 minutes.

6. Season with salt and pepper.

7. Serve hot with a slice of crusty bread.

Spinach in Smoothies

Spinach blends well into smoothies, adding nutrients without over-powering the flavor. Here's a simple smoothie recipe:

Ingredients:

- 1 cup of fresh spinach leaves

- 1 banana

- 1/2 cup of frozen mango chunks

- 1/2 cup of Greek yogurt

- 1 cup of almond milk

- 1 tablespoon of chia seeds (optional)

Instructions:

1. Place all ingredients in a blender.

2. Blend until smooth.

3. Pour into a glass and enjoy immediately.

Spinach Recipes to Try

Here are a few more delicious recipes to help you incorporate spinach into your diet:

Spinach and Cheese Stuffed Chicken Breast

Ingredients:

- 4 boneless, skinless chicken breasts

- 2 cups of fresh spinach leaves, chopped

- 1/2 cup of ricotta cheese

- 1/4 cup of grated Parmesan cheese

- 1 garlic clove, minced

- Salt and pepper to taste

- 2 tablespoons of olive oil

Instructions:

1. Preheat your oven to 375°F (190°C).

2. In a bowl, combine the spinach, ricotta cheese, Parmesan cheese, garlic, salt, and pepper.

3. Cut a pocket into each chicken breast and stuff with the spinach mixture.

4. Heat the olive oil in an oven-safe skillet over medium heat.

5. Sear the chicken breasts on both sides until golden brown.

6. Transfer the skillet to the oven and bake for 20-25 minutes, or until the chicken is cooked through.

7. Serve hot with your favorite side dish.

Spinach and Feta Omelet

Ingredients:

- 3 eggs

- 1/4 cup of fresh spinach leaves, chopped

- 1/4 cup of feta cheese, crumbled

- 1 tablespoon of milk

- 1 tablespoon of olive oil

- Salt and pepper to taste

Instructions:

1. In a bowl, whisk together the eggs and milk.

2. Heat the olive oil in a non-stick skillet over medium heat.

3. Pour the egg mixture into the skillet and cook until the edges start to set.

4. Add the spinach and feta cheese to one half of the omelet.

5. Fold the other half over the filling and cook for another 2-3 minutes, or until the eggs are fully cooked.

6. Season with salt and pepper and serve immediately.

Spinach is a true nutritional powerhouse, offering a wealth of benefits for your bones, digestion, and eyesight. By incorporating spinach into your diet through the practical tips and delicious recipes provided, you can enjoy the many advantages of this nutrient-dense leafy green. The health-boosting power of spinach can transform your diet one delicious meal at a time.

Quinoa

The Complete Protein Powerhouse

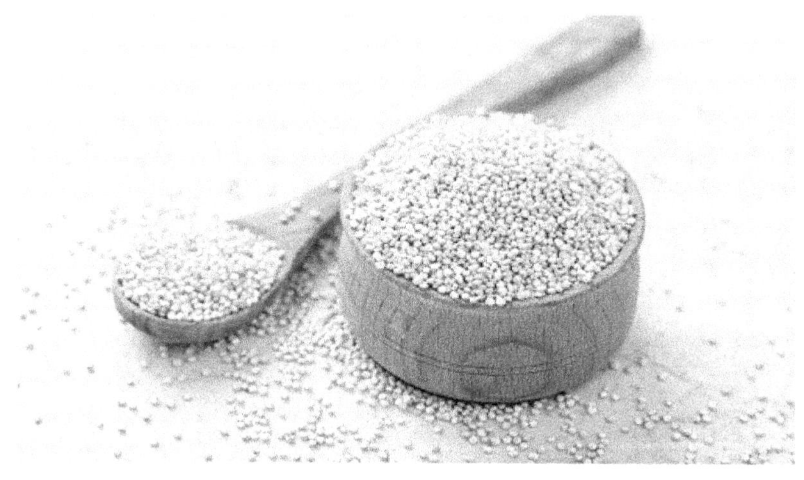

Quinoa, often mistaken for a grain, is actually a seed that has gained immense popularity due to its exceptional nutritional profile. Known as a complete protein, quinoa contains all nine essential amino acids, making it a powerful addition to any diet. This chapter will explore the unique benefits of quinoa, its specific contributions to health and fitness, and provide practical tips and recipes to help you incorporate this nutrient-rich food into your meals.

The Nutritional Profile of Quinoa

Quinoa is a nutritional powerhouse, offering a variety of essential nutrients. A 100-gram serving of cooked quinoa contains:

- Calories: 120

- Protein: 4.1 grams

- Fat: 1.9 grams

- Carbohydrates: 21.3 grams

- Fiber: 2.8 grams

- Vitamin B1 (Thiamine): 10% of the Daily Value (DV)

- Vitamin B2 (Riboflavin): 15% of the DV

- Vitamin B6: 15% of the DV

- Folate: 10% of the DV

- Iron: 8% of the DV

- Magnesium: 16% of the DV

- Manganese: 23% of the DV

In addition to these nutrients, quinoa is gluten-free and rich in antioxidants, making it suitable for a wide range of dietary needs and preferences.

Quinoa and Muscle Repair and Growth

One of the standout benefits of quinoa is its complete protein profile. Here's how quinoa supports muscle repair and growth:

Complete Protein Source

Quinoa is unique among plant-based foods because it contains all nine essential amino acids that the body cannot produce on its own. These amino acids are crucial for muscle repair, growth, and overall health. By providing a complete protein source, quinoa helps meet the protein needs of both vegetarians and omnivores, making it an excellent addition to post-workout meals.

Post-Workout Recovery

After intense exercise, your muscles need protein to repair and grow. Including quinoa in your post-workout meals can help speed up recovery and support muscle development. Its balanced amino acid profile ensures that your body has the necessary building blocks to repair muscle tissue effectively.

Quinoa for Weight Management

Quinoa is also a valuable ally in weight management. Here's how it can help you maintain a healthy body composition:

High in Protein and Fiber

Quinoa's high protein and fiber content can help you feel fuller for longer, promoting satiety and preventing overeating. Protein is known for its ability to reduce hunger and increase feelings of fullness, while fiber adds bulk to your meals and slows down digestion. Together, these nutrients can help you control your appetite and manage your weight more effectively.

Low Glycemic Index

Quinoa has a low glycemic index, meaning it causes a slower, more gradual rise in blood sugar levels compared to refined carbohydrates. This helps prevent spikes and crashes in blood sugar, reducing cravings and supporting better weight management.

Sustained Energy from Quinoa

Quinoa provides sustained energy throughout the day, making it an excellent choice for busy schedules and intense workouts. Here's how it works:

Complex Carbohydrates

Unlike refined carbohydrates, quinoa is a complex carbohydrate that is digested slowly. This slow digestion releases energy steadily, helping to keep you energized and focused for longer periods. Quinoa's complex carbohydrates are particularly beneficial for athletes and those with demanding daily routines.

Nutrient-Rich Fuel

In addition to providing sustained energy, quinoa offers a range of essential nutrients that support overall health and well-being. Its combination of protein, fiber, vitamins, and minerals makes it a nutrient-dense choice for fueling your body.

Delicious Ways to Enjoy Quinoa

Quinoa's versatility makes it easy to incorporate into your meals. Here are some delicious ways to enjoy this nutrient-rich food:

Quinoa Salads and Grain Bowls

Quinoa makes a fantastic base for salads and grain bowls. Here's a simple quinoa salad recipe:

Ingredients:

- 1 cup of cooked quinoa

- 1 cup of cherry tomatoes, halved

- 1 cucumber, diced

- 1/4 cup of red onion, finely chopped

- 1/4 cup of feta cheese, crumbled

- 2 tablespoons of olive oil

- Juice of 1 lemon

- Salt and pepper to taste

Instructions:

1. In a large bowl, combine the cooked quinoa, cherry tomatoes, cucumber, red onion, and feta cheese.

2. Drizzle with olive oil and lemon juice.

3. Season with salt and pepper, then toss to combine.

4. Serve chilled or at room temperature.

Quinoa as a Side Dish

Quinoa can be used as a nutritious side dish instead of rice or pasta. Here's a basic recipe:

Ingredients:

- 1 cup of quinoa

- 2 cups of water or vegetable broth

- 1 tablespoon of olive oil

- Salt to taste

Instructions:

1. Rinse the quinoa under cold water.

2. In a medium saucepan, bring the water or vegetable broth to a boil.

3. Add the quinoa, reduce heat to low, and cover.

4. Simmer for 15-20 minutes, or until the quinoa is tender and the liquid is absorbed.

5. Fluff with a fork and drizzle with olive oil.

6. Season with salt and serve as a side dish.

Quinoa in Soups and Stews

Adding quinoa to soups and stews is an easy way to boost their protein and texture. Here's a hearty quinoa soup recipe:

Ingredients:

- 1 tablespoon of olive oil

- 1 onion, chopped

- 2 garlic cloves, minced

- 2 carrots, sliced

- 2 celery stalks, sliced

- 1 cup of cooked quinoa

- 4 cups of vegetable broth

- 1 can of diced tomatoes

- 1 teaspoon of dried thyme

- 1 teaspoon of dried basil

- Salt and pepper to taste

Instructions:

1. Heat the olive oil in a large pot over medium heat.

2. Add the onion, garlic, carrots, and celery, and sauté until the vegetables are tender.

3. Stir in the vegetable broth, diced tomatoes, thyme, and basil.

4. Bring to a boil, then reduce heat and simmer for 20 minutes.

5. Add the cooked quinoa and cook for an additional 5 minutes.

6. Season with salt and pepper, then serve hot.

Quinoa Recipes to Try

Here are a few more delicious recipes to help you incorporate quinoa into your diet:

Quinoa and Black Bean Stuffed Peppers

Ingredients:

- 4 bell peppers, tops cut off and seeds removed

- 1 cup of cooked quinoa

- 1 can of black beans, drained and rinsed

- 1 cup of corn kernels

- 1/2 cup of salsa

- 1 teaspoon of cumin

- 1/2 teaspoon of chili powder

- 1/4 cup of shredded cheese (optional)

Instructions:

1. Preheat your oven to 375°F (190°C).

2. In a large bowl, combine the cooked quinoa, black beans, corn, salsa, cumin, and chili powder.

3. Stuff the mixture into the bell peppers.

4. Place the stuffed peppers in a baking dish and cover with foil.

5. Bake for 30 minutes, then remove the foil and sprinkle with cheese, if using.

6. Bake for an additional 10 minutes, or until the peppers are tender.

7. Serve hot.

Quinoa Breakfast Porridge

Ingredients:

- 1 cup of cooked quinoa

- 1 cup of almond milk or any milk of your choice

- 1 tablespoon of honey or maple syrup

- 1/2 teaspoon of cinnamon

- Fresh berries or sliced fruit for topping

Instructions:

1. In a medium saucepan, combine the cooked quinoa, almond milk, honey, and cinnamon.

2. Bring to a simmer over medium heat, stirring occasionally.

3. Cook for 5-7 minutes, or until the mixture thickens to your desired consistency.

4. Serve warm, topped with fresh berries or sliced fruit.

Quinoa is an exceptional source of complete protein, offering numerous health benefits including muscle repair and growth, weight management, and sustained energy. By incorporating quinoa into your diet through the practical tips and delicious recipes provided, you can enjoy the many advantages of this nutrient-rich seed. The power of quinoa can transform your health one flavorful meal at a time.

Make a Difference with Your Review

Unlock the Power of Generosity

> *"Helping one person might not change the whole world, but it could change the world for one person." - Unknown*

People who give without expectation live longer, happier lives and make more money. So if we've got a shot at that during our time together, darn it, I'm gonna try.

To make it happen, I have a simple question for you...

Would you lend a helping hand to someone you've never met, even if you never got credit for it? Who is this person, you ask?

They are just like you once were—eager to learn, looking for guidance, and wanting to make positive changes in their eating habits but unsure where to start.

My mission is to make healthy eating accessible to everyone. And the only way to reach this goal is by connecting with as many people as possible.

This is where you come in. Most people do, in fact, judge a book by its cover (and its reviews). So here's my request on behalf of a health-conscious person you've never met:

Please help that reader by leaving a review for this book. Your gift costs no money and takes less than 60 seconds to give, but it can change a fellow healthy food option seeker's life forever.

Your review could help...

...one more health-conscious person discover the power of superfoods.

...one more family start eating healthier.

...one more community embrace better nutrition.

...one more dream come true.

To get that 'feel good' feeling and help this person for real, all you have to do is...and it takes less than 60 seconds...leave a review.

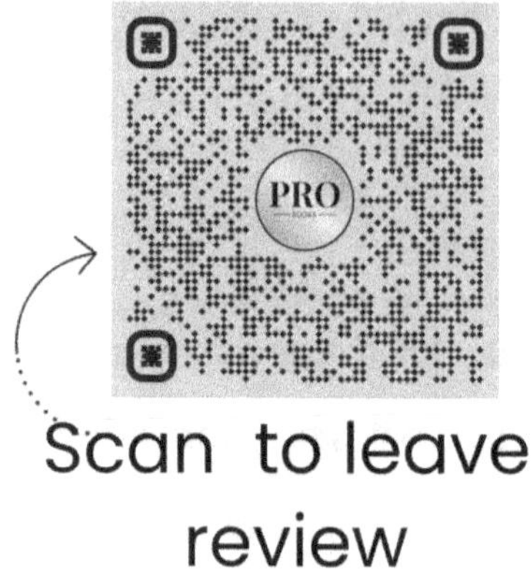

If you feel good about helping a faceless reader, you are my kind of person. Welcome to the club. You're one of us.

I'm that much more excited to help you transform your health with nature's best nutrient-rich foods faster and easier than you can possibly imagine. You'll love the tips and recipes I'm about to share in the coming chapters.

Thank you from the bottom of my heart. Now, back to our regularly scheduled programming.

-Your biggest fan, Conard

PS - Fun fact: If you provide something of value to another person, it makes you more valuable to them. If you believe this book will help someone you know, send it their way.

Avocado

The Healthy Fat Superstar

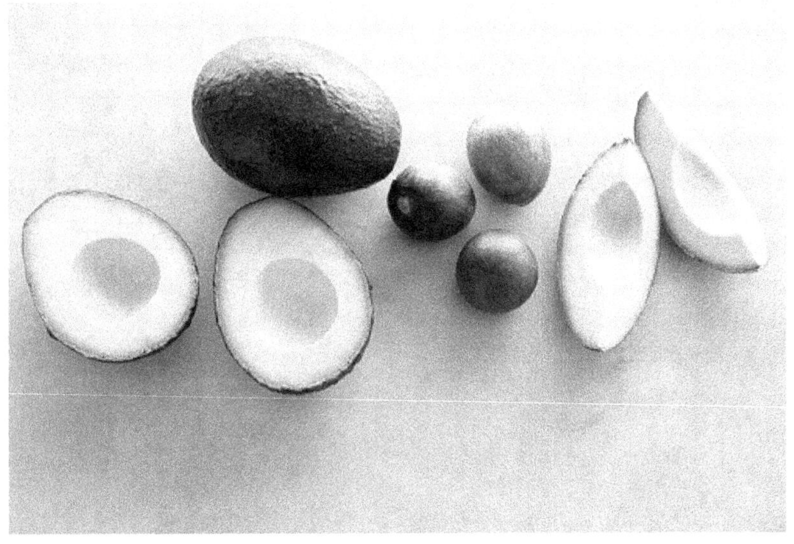

Avocados, often hailed as a superfood, are celebrated for their creamy texture and rich nutritional profile. Packed with heart-healthy monounsaturated fats and essential nutrients like potassium, avocados offer a range of health benefits that make them a valuable addition to any diet. In this chapter, we will explore the numerous health benefits of avocados, delve into their specific contributions to overall well-being, and provide practical tips and recipes to help you incorporate this versatile fruit into your daily meals.

The Nutritional Profile of Avocado

Avocados are nutrient-dense, providing a variety of essential vitamins, minerals, and healthy fats. A 100-gram serving of avocado contains:

- Calories: 160

- Fat: 15 grams (of which 10 grams are monounsaturated)

- Carbohydrates: 9 grams

- Fiber: 7 grams

- Protein: 2 grams

- Vitamin K: 26% of the Daily Value (DV)

- Folate: 20% of the DV

- Vitamin C: 17% of the DV

- Potassium: 14% of the DV

- Vitamin E: 10% of the DV

In addition to these nutrients, avocados are rich in antioxidants, including lutein and zeaxanthin, which contribute to their health-promoting properties.

Avocado Supports Heart Health

Avocados are renowned for their heart-healthy benefits. Here's how they support cardiovascular health:

Monounsaturated Fats

The majority of the fat in avocados is monounsaturated fat, which is known to improve heart health by lowering levels of bad LDL cholesterol while increasing good HDL cholesterol. This balance helps reduce the risk of heart disease and stroke.

Potassium Content

Avocados are an excellent source of potassium, an essential mineral that helps regulate blood pressure. Adequate potassium intake can help counteract the effects of sodium and reduce hypertension, further supporting heart health.

Improved Digestion with Avocado

Avocados are a digestive superstar thanks to their high fiber content. Here's how they promote digestive health:

Fiber for Digestive Health

One of the standout features of avocados is their fiber content, with both soluble and insoluble fiber present. Soluble fiber helps feed the beneficial bacteria in your gut, promoting a healthy microbiome, while insoluble fiber adds bulk to your stool and aids in regular bowel movements, preventing constipation and promoting overall digestive health.

Improve Your Skin's Appearance with Avocado

The combination of healthy fats and antioxidants in avocados makes them a beauty booster from the inside out. Here's how avocados enhance skin health:

Hydration and Elasticity

The healthy fats in avocados help keep your skin hydrated and supple. These fats maintain the skin's moisture barrier, preventing dryness and improving skin elasticity, which can reduce the appearance of fine lines and wrinkles.

Antioxidant Protection

Avocados are rich in antioxidants like vitamins C and E, which protect the skin from oxidative damage caused by free radicals. This protection helps keep the skin looking youthful and vibrant while promoting an even skin tone.

Delicious Ways to Enjoy Avocado

Incorporating avocados into your diet can be both easy and delicious. Here are some creative ways to enjoy this nutrient-rich fruit:

Avocado Toast

Avocado toast is a simple and nutritious way to start your day. Here's a basic recipe:

Ingredients:

- 1 ripe avocado

- 2 slices of whole-grain bread

- Salt and pepper to taste

- Optional toppings: cherry tomatoes, feta cheese, red pepper flakes, poached egg

Instructions:

1. Toast the slices of whole-grain bread to your desired level of crispiness.

2. While the bread is toasting, scoop out the flesh of the avocado into a bowl.

3. Mash the avocado with a fork until it reaches your preferred consistency.

4. Spread the mashed avocado evenly onto the toasted bread.

5. Season with salt and pepper.

6. Add any optional toppings, such as cherry tomatoes, feta cheese, red pepper flakes, or a poached egg.

7. Serve immediately and enjoy.

Avocado in Salads and Sandwiches

Adding sliced avocado to salads and sandwiches provides extra creaminess and flavor. Here's a simple salad recipe:

Ingredients:

- 4 cups of mixed greens

- 1 ripe avocado, sliced

- 1/2 cup of cherry tomatoes, halved

- 1/4 cup of red onion, thinly sliced

- 1/4 cup of feta cheese, crumbled

- 2 tablespoons of olive oil

- Juice of 1 lemon

- Salt and pepper to taste

Instructions:

1. In a large bowl, combine the mixed greens, sliced avocado, cherry tomatoes, red onion, and feta cheese.

2. Drizzle with olive oil and lemon juice.

3. Season with salt and pepper, then toss to combine.

4. Serve immediately as a refreshing and nutritious salad.

Avocado Smoothies

Blending avocado into smoothies adds a creamy texture and a boost of nutrients. Here's a simple avocado smoothie recipe:

Ingredients:

- 1 ripe avocado

- 1 banana

- 1 cup of spinach leaves

- 1 cup of almond milk or any milk of your choice

- 1 tablespoon of honey or maple syrup (optional)

- Ice cubes (optional)

Instructions:

1. Place all ingredients in a blender.

2. Blend until smooth and creamy.

3. Add ice cubes if desired and blend again.

4. Pour into a glass and enjoy immediately.

Avocado Recipes to Try

Here are a few more delicious recipes to help you incorporate avocado into your diet:

Guacamole

Ingredients:

- 2 ripe avocados

- 1 small red onion, finely chopped

- 1-2 cloves of garlic, minced

- 1-2 tomatoes, diced

- Juice of 1 lime

- Salt and pepper to taste

- Optional: chopped cilantro, jalapeño, or cumin

Instructions:

1. Cut the avocados in half, remove the pits, and scoop out the flesh into a bowl.

2. Mash the avocado with a fork until it reaches your desired consistency.

3. Stir in the chopped red onion, garlic, and tomatoes.

4. Add lime juice and season with salt and pepper.

5. Mix in any optional ingredients, such as cilantro, jalapeño, or cumin.

6. Serve immediately with tortilla chips or as a topping for tacos and other dishes.

Avocado Egg Salad

Ingredients:

- 4 hard-boiled eggs, chopped

- 1 ripe avocado, diced

- 2 tablespoons of Greek yogurt or mayonnaise

- 1 teaspoon of Dijon mustard

- 1 tablespoon of fresh chives, chopped

- Salt and pepper to taste

Instructions:

1. In a large bowl, combine the chopped hard-boiled eggs and diced avocado.

2. Add the Greek yogurt or mayonnaise and Dijon mustard.

3. Stir in the chopped chives and season with salt and pepper.

4. Mix until well combined.

5. Serve as a sandwich filling, on toast, or with crackers.

Avocados are more than just a delicious addition to your meals; they are a nutritional powerhouse that supports heart health, improves digestion, and enhances skin health. By incorporating avocados into your diet through the practical tips and delicious recipes provided, you can enjoy the many advantages of this healthy fat superstar. The creamy, nutritious goodness of avocados can transform your health one tasty bite at a time.

Chapter Seven

Chia Seeds

The Tiny Nutritional Powerhouses

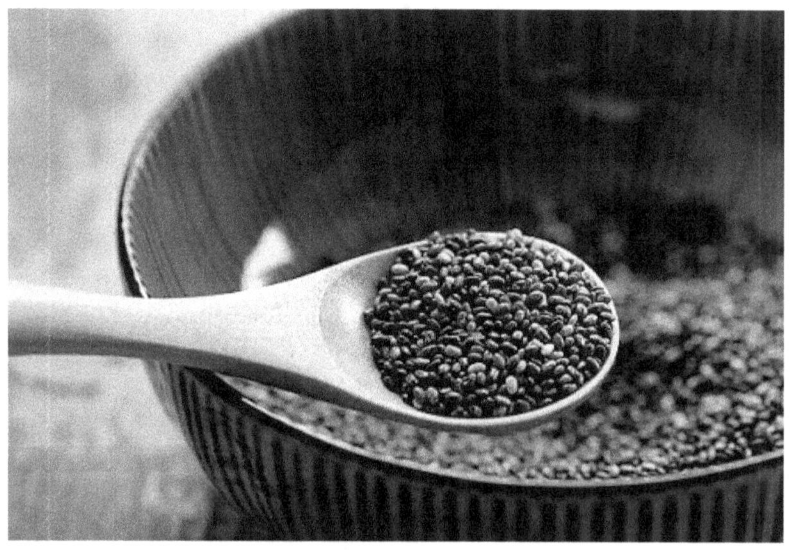

Chia seeds may be small, but they are packed with nutrients that provide a myriad of health benefits. These tiny seeds, derived from the Salvia hispanica plant, have gained popularity for their high fiber content, omega-3 fatty acids, and powerful antioxidants. In this chapter, we will explore the health benefits of chia seeds, how they can support various aspects of health, and provide practical tips and recipes to incorporate these versatile seeds into your daily diet.

The Nutritional Profile of Chia Seeds

Chia seeds are incredibly nutrient-dense, offering a range of essential vitamins, minerals, and other beneficial compounds. A 28-gram (1-ounce) serving of chia seeds contains:

- Calories: 137

- Protein: 4 grams

- Fat: 9 grams (including 5 grams of omega-3 fatty acids)

- Carbohydrates: 12 grams

- Fiber: 11 grams

- Calcium: 18% of the Daily Value (DV)

- Manganese: 30% of the DV

- Phosphorus: 27% of the DV

In addition to these nutrients, chia seeds are rich in antioxidants, which help protect the body from oxidative stress and inflammation.

Promotes Digestive Health with Chia Seeds

One of the standout benefits of chia seeds is their high fiber content, which promotes digestive health. Here's how chia seeds support your digestive system:

High Fiber Content

Chia seeds are an excellent source of dietary fiber, with most of it being soluble fiber. This type of fiber absorbs water and forms a gel-like substance in the digestive tract, adding bulk to the stool and helping it move smoothly through the intestines. This process can prevent constipation, promote regular bowel movements, and maintain overall digestive health.

Prebiotic Properties

The fiber in chia seeds also acts as a prebiotic, feeding the beneficial bacteria in your gut. A healthy gut microbiome is essential for optimal digestion, immune function, and overall health. By supporting the growth of good bacteria, chia seeds contribute to a balanced and healthy digestive system.

Aids in Weight Loss with Chia Seeds

Chia seeds can be a valuable ally in weight management. Here's how they help:

Satiety and Fullness

Despite their small size, chia seeds are highly effective at promoting satiety. When mixed with liquid, chia seeds expand and form a gel-like substance in the stomach, which can help you feel full and satisfied for longer periods. This increased feeling of fullness can curb cravings and reduce overall calorie intake, making chia seeds a helpful addition to weight loss efforts.

Low in Calories

Chia seeds are nutrient-dense but relatively low in calories, allowing you to add them to meals and snacks without significantly increasing your caloric intake. This makes them an excellent option for those looking to manage their weight while still getting essential nutrients.

Helps Regulate Blood Sugar Levels with Chia Seeds

The combination of fiber and omega-3 fatty acids in chia seeds can help stabilize blood sugar levels. Here's how:

Slowing Carbohydrate Absorption

The soluble fiber in chia seeds slows the digestion and absorption of carbohydrates, leading to a more gradual release of glucose into the bloodstream. This helps prevent spikes and crashes in blood sugar levels, which can lead to energy slumps and cravings.

Omega-3 Fatty Acids

Omega-3 fatty acids in chia seeds have anti-inflammatory properties that can help improve insulin sensitivity. Better insulin sensitivity allows the body to use glucose more effectively, reducing the risk of type 2 diabetes and helping to maintain stable blood sugar levels.

Delicious Ways to Enjoy Chia Seeds

Incorporating chia seeds into your diet is easy and versatile. Here are some delicious ways to enjoy these tiny nutritional powerhouses:

Chia Seed Pudding

Chia seed pudding is a simple and nutritious way to enjoy chia seeds. Here's a basic recipe:

Ingredients:

- 1/4 cup of chia seeds

- 1 cup of almond milk or any milk of your choice

- 1 tablespoon of honey or maple syrup

- 1/2 teaspoon of vanilla extract

Instructions:

1. In a bowl, combine the chia seeds, almond milk, honey, and vanilla extract.

2. Stir well to combine.

3. Let the mixture sit for 5 minutes, then stir again to break up any clumps.

4. Cover and refrigerate for at least 2 hours, or overnight, until it reaches a pudding-like consistency.

5. Serve with your favorite toppings, such as fresh fruit, nuts, or granola.

Chia Seed Smoothies

Adding chia seeds to smoothies is an easy way to boost their nutritional content. Here's a simple smoothie recipe:

Ingredients:

- 1 cup of spinach leaves

- 1 banana

- 1/2 cup of frozen berries

- 1 tablespoon of chia seeds

- 1 cup of almond milk or any milk of your choice

- 1 tablespoon of honey or maple syrup (optional)

Instructions:

1. Place all ingredients in a blender.

2. Blend until smooth.

3. Pour into a glass and enjoy immediately.

Chia Seed Energy Bars

Homemade chia seed energy bars are a convenient and healthy snack. Here's a recipe to try:

Ingredients:

- 1 cup of rolled oats

- 1/2 cup of almond butter

- 1/4 cup of honey or maple syrup

- 1/4 cup of chia seeds

- 1/4 cup of dried fruit, chopped (e.g., cranberries, apricots)

- 1/4 cup of nuts, chopped (e.g., almonds, walnuts)

Instructions:

1. In a large bowl, combine the rolled oats, chia seeds, dried fruit, and nuts.

2. In a microwave-safe bowl, heat the almond butter and honey for 20-30 seconds, or until melted and easy to mix.

3. Pour the almond butter mixture over the dry ingredients and stir until well combined.

4. Press the mixture into a parchment-lined baking dish.

5. Refrigerate for at least 1 hour, or until firm.

6. Cut into bars and store in an airtight container in the refrigerator.

Chia seeds are small but mighty, offering a wealth of health benefits including improved digestive health, weight loss support, and blood sugar regulation. By incorporating chia seeds into your diet through the practical tips and delicious recipes provided, you can enjoy the many advantages of these tiny nutritional powerhouses. The impressive nutrient profile of chia seeds can transform your health one small seed at a time.

Chapter Eight

Broccoli

The Nutrient-Packed Veggie

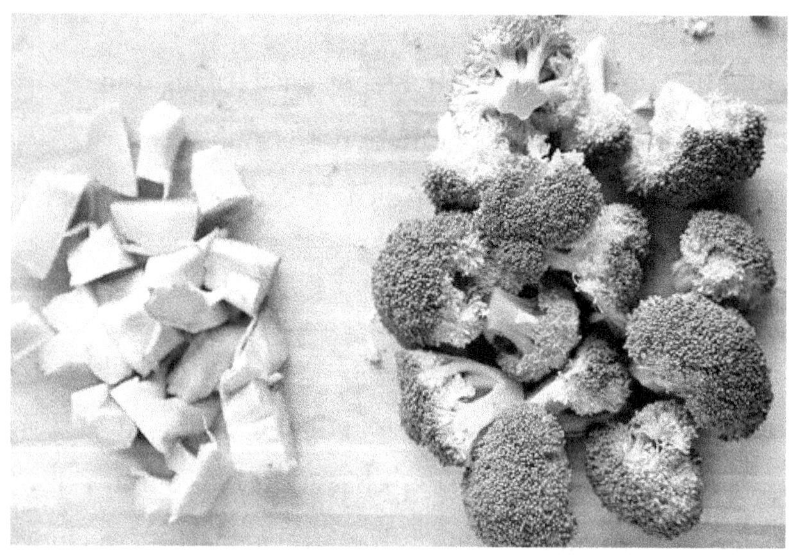

Broccoli is more than just a green vegetable; it's a nutritional powerhouse that can significantly enhance your health. Packed with essential vitamins, minerals, and fiber, broccoli offers a variety of health benefits. In this chapter, we will explore the numerous advantages of incorporating broccoli into your diet, delve into the science behind its health benefits, and provide practical tips and recipes to help you enjoy this versatile vegetable in your daily meals.

The Nutritional Profile of Broccoli

Broccoli is loaded with nutrients that are vital for maintaining good health. A 100-gram serving of raw broccoli contains:

- Calories: 34

- Protein: 2.8 grams

- Carbohydrates: 6.6 grams

- Fiber: 2.6 grams

- Vitamin C: 89% of the Daily Value (DV)

- Vitamin K: 85% of the DV

- Folate: 16% of the DV

- Potassium: 8% of the DV

- Vitamin A: 12% of the DV

In addition to these nutrients, broccoli is rich in antioxidants and phytochemicals, which contribute to its health-promoting properties.

Supports Detoxification with Broccoli

One of the key benefits of broccoli is its ability to support the body's natural detoxification processes. Here's how it works:

Glucosinolates and Detoxification

Broccoli contains compounds called glucosinolates, which play a crucial role in the body's detoxification system. When you consume broccoli, these glucosinolates are broken down into active compounds like sulforaphane and indole-3-carbinol. These compounds enhance the liver's ability to detoxify harmful substances and eliminate them from the body.

Enhancing Phase II Detoxification

The compounds in broccoli support phase II detoxification enzymes in the liver, which are responsible for neutralizing and excreting toxins. By boosting these enzymes, broccoli helps the body efficiently detoxify and protect against environmental pollutants, harmful chemicals, and metabolic byproducts.

Boosts Immunity with Broccoli

Broccoli is a fantastic food for boosting your immune system, thanks to its high vitamin C content and other immune-supporting nutrients.

Vitamin C and Immune Function

Vitamin C is essential for the proper functioning of the immune system. It helps stimulate the production of white blood cells, which are crucial for fighting infections. Additionally, vitamin C acts as an antioxidant, protecting immune cells from damage caused by free radicals.

Antioxidant Support

Beyond vitamin C, broccoli contains other antioxidants like beta-carotene, selenium, and vitamin E. These antioxidants work together to strengthen the immune system, reduce inflammation, and enhance the body's ability to fend off illnesses.

May Reduce the Risk of Certain Cancers with Broccoli

Broccoli belongs to the cruciferous vegetable family, which is known for its cancer-fighting properties. Here's how broccoli can help reduce the risk of certain cancers:

Cancer-Fighting Compounds

The glucosinolates in broccoli are converted into compounds that have been shown to inhibit the growth of cancer cells and promote their destruction. Sulforaphane, in particular, has been extensively studied for its anti-cancer properties. It helps deactivate carcinogens, reduce inflammation, and prevent the growth and spread of cancer cells.

Supporting Cellular Health

Broccoli's combination of antioxidants, vitamins, and minerals supports overall cellular health. By protecting cells from oxidative damage and enhancing DNA repair, broccoli helps maintain the integrity of healthy cells and reduce the risk of cancer development.

Delicious Ways to Enjoy Broccoli

Incorporating broccoli into your diet can be both easy and delicious. Here are some creative ways to enjoy this nutrient-packed vegetable:

Steamed or Roasted Broccoli

Steaming or roasting broccoli is a simple and nutritious way to prepare it. Here's a basic recipe for roasted broccoli:

Ingredients:

- 1 head of broccoli, cut into florets

- 2 tablespoons of olive oil

- 2 cloves of garlic, minced

- Salt and pepper to taste

- Lemon juice (optional)

Instructions:

1. Preheat your oven to 425°F (220°C).

2. In a large bowl, toss the broccoli florets with olive oil, minced garlic, salt, and pepper.

3. Spread the broccoli in a single layer on a baking sheet.

4. Roast for 20-25 minutes, or until the broccoli is tender and slightly crispy on the edges.

5. Squeeze fresh lemon juice over the roasted broccoli before serving, if desired.

Broccoli in Stir-Fries and Pasta

Adding broccoli to stir-fries and pasta dishes is an excellent way to boost their nutritional content. Here's a simple broccoli stir-fry recipe:

Ingredients:

- 2 tablespoons of olive oil

- 1 head of broccoli, cut into florets

- 1 red bell pepper, sliced

- 1 carrot, julienned

- 2 cloves of garlic, minced

- 2 tablespoons of soy sauce

- 1 tablespoon of oyster sauce

- 1 teaspoon of sesame oil

- Cooked rice or noodles for serving

Instructions:

1. Heat the olive oil in a large skillet or wok over medium-high heat.

2. Add the garlic and sauté for 30 seconds, until fragrant.

3. Add the broccoli, bell pepper, and carrot to the skillet.

4. Stir-fry for 5-7 minutes, or until the vegetables are tender-crisp.

5. Add the soy sauce, oyster sauce, and sesame oil, and stir to combine.

6. Serve the stir-fry over cooked rice or noodles.

Raw Broccoli in Salads

Enjoying broccoli raw in salads provides a crunchy texture and fresh flavor. Here's a simple broccoli salad recipe:

Ingredients:

- 4 cups of raw broccoli florets

- 1/4 cup of red onion, finely chopped

- 1/4 cup of dried cranberries

- 1/4 cup of sunflower seeds

- 1/2 cup of Greek yogurt

- 2 tablespoons of apple cider vinegar

- 1 tablespoon of honey

- Salt and pepper to taste

Instructions:

1. In a large bowl, combine the broccoli florets, red onion, dried cranberries, and sunflower seeds.

2. In a small bowl, whisk together the Greek yogurt, apple cider vinegar, honey, salt, and pepper.

3. Pour the dressing over the broccoli mixture and toss to coat.

4. Serve immediately or refrigerate until ready to eat.

Broccoli Recipes to Try

Here are a few more delicious recipes to help you incorporate broccoli into your diet:

Broccoli Cheddar Soup

Ingredients:

- 2 tablespoons of butter

- 1 onion, chopped

- 2 cloves of garlic, minced

- 1 head of broccoli, cut into florets

- 4 cups of vegetable broth

- 1 cup of shredded cheddar cheese

- 1/2 cup of milk or cream

- Salt and pepper to taste

Instructions:

1. In a large pot, melt the butter over medium heat.

2. Add the onion and garlic, and sauté until the onion is translucent.

3. Add the broccoli and vegetable broth, and bring to a boil.

4. Reduce heat and simmer for 10-15 minutes, or until the broccoli is tender.

5. Using an immersion blender, blend the soup until smooth.

6. Stir in the shredded cheddar cheese and milk or cream.

7. Season with salt and pepper.

8. Serve hot with a crusty bread.

Broccoli and Quinoa Salad

Ingredients:

- 1 cup of cooked quinoa

- 1 head of broccoli, cut into florets and steamed

- 1/2 cup of cherry tomatoes, halved

- 1/4 cup of red onion, finely chopped

- 1/4 cup of feta cheese, crumbled

- 2 tablespoons of olive oil

- Juice of 1 lemon

- Salt and pepper to taste

Instructions:

1. In a large bowl, combine the cooked quinoa, steamed broccoli, cherry tomatoes, red onion, and feta cheese.

2. Drizzle with olive oil and lemon juice.

3. Season with salt and pepper, then toss to combine.

4. Serve chilled or at room temperature.

Broccoli is a nutritional powerhouse that supports detoxification, boosts immunity, and may reduce the risk of certain cancers. By incorporating broccoli into your diet through the practical tips and delicious recipes provided, you can enjoy the many advantages of this versatile vegetable. The health benefits of broccoli can transform your diet one delicious meal at a time.

Chapter Nine

Sweet Potatoes

The Nutrient-Packed Tubers

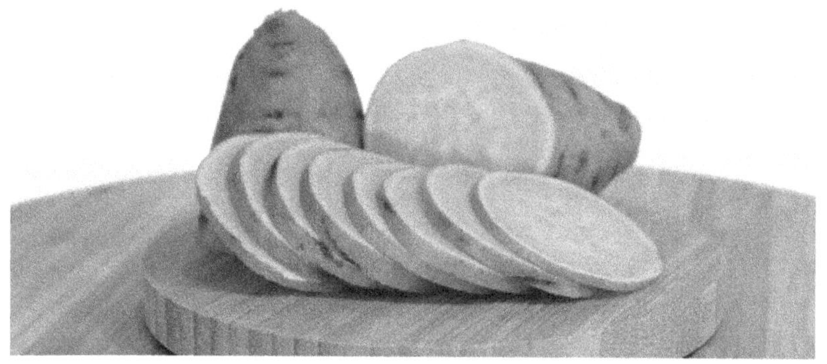

Sweet potatoes, with their vibrant orange hue and natural sweetness, are more than just a delicious treat. These nutrient-packed tubers are rich in essential vitamins, minerals, fiber, and antioxidants, making them a powerhouse of nutrition. This chapter will explore the numerous health benefits of sweet potatoes, delve into their specific contributions to overall well-being, and provide practical tips and recipes to help you incorporate this versatile food into your daily meals.

The Nutritional Profile of Sweet Potatoes

Sweet potatoes are incredibly nutrient-dense, providing a variety of essential vitamins and minerals. A 100-gram serving of baked sweet potato with skin contains:

- Calories: 90

- Protein: 2 grams

- Fat: 0.15 grams

- Carbohydrates: 21 grams

- Fiber: 3 grams

- Vitamin A: 283% of the Daily Value (DV)

- Vitamin C: 32% of the DV

- Manganese: 14% of the DV

- Potassium: 10% of the DV

- Vitamin B6: 10% of the DV

In addition to these nutrients, sweet potatoes are rich in antioxidants like beta-carotene, which contributes to their vibrant color and numerous health benefits.

Sweet Potatoes for your Eyes

One of the standout benefits of sweet potatoes is their ability to support and enhance eye health. Here's how they work:

Vitamin A and Vision

Sweet potatoes are an excellent source of vitamin A, primarily in the form of beta-carotene, which is converted into vitamin A in the body. Vitamin A is crucial for maintaining good vision, particularly in low-light conditions. It helps protect the surface of the eye and contributes to the health of the cornea and conjunctiva. Regular consumption of sweet potatoes can help prevent vitamin A deficiency, which is a leading cause of preventable blindness in children.

Antioxidant Protection

The antioxidants in sweet potatoes, including beta-carotene and vitamin C, help protect the eyes from oxidative stress and damage caused by free radicals. This protection can reduce the risk of age-related macular degeneration (AMD) and cataracts, keeping your vision sharp and healthy as you age.

Boosts Immunity with Sweet Potatoes

Sweet potatoes are a fantastic food for boosting your immune system, thanks to their high vitamin C content and other immune-supporting nutrients.

Vitamin C and Immune Function

Vitamin C is essential for the proper functioning of the immune system. It stimulates the production of white blood cells, which are crucial for fighting infections. Additionally, vitamin C acts as an antioxidant, protecting immune cells from damage caused by free radicals. Consuming sweet potatoes regularly can help strengthen your immune system and make you less susceptible to colds, flu, and other infections.

Anti-inflammatory Properties

Sweet potatoes contain various compounds with anti-inflammatory properties, such as beta-carotene and other antioxidants. These compounds help reduce inflammation in the body, supporting overall immune health and reducing the risk of chronic diseases.

Helps Regulate Blood Sugar Levels with Sweet Potatoes

Despite their natural sweetness, sweet potatoes have a low glycemic index (GI), making them a diabetic-friendly food choice. Here's how they help regulate blood sugar levels:

Low Glycemic Index

The glycemic index measures how quickly a food raises blood sugar levels. Foods with a low GI, like sweet potatoes, are digested and absorbed more slowly, causing a gradual rise in blood sugar rather than a rapid spike. This slow release of sugar into the bloodstream helps maintain stable blood sugar levels, which is beneficial for people with diabetes and those looking to manage their weight.

High Fiber Content

The fiber in sweet potatoes plays a crucial role in regulating blood sugar levels. Fiber slows down the absorption of sugar in the digestive tract, preventing spikes and crashes in blood sugar. This helps keep energy levels stable and reduces the risk of insulin resistance and type 2 diabetes.

Delicious Ways to Enjoy Sweet Potatoes

Incorporating sweet potatoes into your diet can be both easy and delicious. Here are some creative ways to enjoy these nutrient-packed tubers:

Roasted Sweet Potato Wedges

Roasting sweet potato wedges is a simple and flavorful way to enjoy this versatile vegetable. Here's a basic recipe:

Ingredients:

- 2 large sweet potatoes, cut into wedges

- 2 tablespoons of olive oil

- 1 teaspoon of paprika

- 1/2 teaspoon of garlic powder

- Salt and pepper to taste

- Fresh parsley for garnish (optional)

Instructions:

1. Preheat your oven to 425°F (220°C).

2. In a large bowl, toss the sweet potato wedges with olive oil, paprika, garlic powder, salt, and pepper.

3. Spread the wedges in a single layer on a baking sheet.

4. Roast for 25-30 minutes, turning halfway through, until the wedges are tender and golden brown.

5. Garnish with fresh parsley before serving, if desired.

Mashed Sweet Potatoes

Mashed sweet potatoes are a delicious and healthier alternative to traditional mashed potatoes. Here's a simple recipe:

Ingredients:

- 4 large sweet potatoes, peeled and cubed

- 2 tablespoons of butter

- 1/4 cup of milk or cream

- 1/2 teaspoon of cinnamon

- 1/4 teaspoon of nutmeg

- Salt to taste

Instructions:

1. Bring a large pot of salted water to a boil.

2. Add the sweet potatoes and cook until tender, about 15-20 minutes.

3. Drain the sweet potatoes and return them to the pot.

4. Add the butter, milk or cream, cinnamon, nutmeg, and salt.

5. Mash the sweet potatoes until smooth and creamy.

6. Serve warm as a side dish.

Sweet Potato Soup

Adding sweet potatoes to soups is an excellent way to boost their nutritional content. Here's a hearty sweet potato soup recipe:

Ingredients:

- 2 tablespoons of olive oil

- 1 onion, chopped

- 2 cloves of garlic, minced

- 2 large sweet potatoes, peeled and diced

- 4 cups of vegetable broth

- 1 teaspoon of ground cumin

- 1/2 teaspoon of smoked paprika

- Salt and pepper to taste

- Fresh cilantro for garnish (optional)

Instructions:

1. Heat the olive oil in a large pot over medium heat.

2. Add the onion and garlic, and sauté until the onion is translucent.

3. Add the sweet potatoes, vegetable broth, cumin, and smoked paprika.

4. Bring to a boil, then reduce heat and simmer for 20-25 minutes, or until the sweet potatoes are tender.

5. Using an immersion blender, blend the soup until smooth.

6. Season with salt and pepper.

7. Garnish with fresh cilantro before serving, if desired.

Sweet Potato Recipes to Try

Here are a few more delicious recipes to help you incorporate sweet potatoes into your diet:

Sweet Potato and Black Bean Chili

Ingredients:

- 1 tablespoon of olive oil

- 1 onion, chopped

- 2 cloves of garlic, minced

- 1 bell pepper, chopped

- 2 large sweet potatoes, peeled and diced

- 1 can of black beans, drained and rinsed

- 1 can of diced tomatoes

- 2 cups of vegetable broth

- 1 tablespoon of chili powder

- 1 teaspoon of ground cumin

- Salt and pepper to taste

Instructions:

1. Heat the olive oil in a large pot over medium heat.

2. Add the onion, garlic, and bell pepper, and sauté until the vegetables are tender.

3. Add the sweet potatoes, black beans, diced tomatoes, vegetable broth, chili powder, and cumin.

4. Bring to a boil, then reduce heat and simmer for 30-35 minutes, or until the sweet potatoes are tender.

5. Season with salt and pepper.

6. Serve hot with your favorite toppings, such as avocado, cilantro, or shredded cheese.

Baked Sweet Potato Fries

Ingredients:

- 2 large sweet potatoes, cut into fries

- 2 tablespoons of olive oil

- 1 teaspoon of paprika

- 1/2 teaspoon of garlic powder

- Salt and pepper to taste

Instructions:

1. Preheat your oven to 425°F (220°C).

2. In a large bowl, toss the sweet potato fries with olive oil,

paprika, garlic powder, salt, and pepper.

3. Spread the fries in a single layer on a baking sheet.

4. Bake for 20-25 minutes, turning halfway through, until the fries are crispy and golden brown.

5. Serve hot with your favorite dipping sauce.

Sweet potatoes are a nutrient-rich food that supports eye health, boosts immunity, and helps regulate blood sugar levels. By incorporating sweet potatoes into your diet through the practical tips and delicious recipes provided, you can enjoy the many advantages of these versatile tubers. Embrace the health benefits of sweet potatoes and transform your diet one flavorful meal at a time.

Chapter Ten

Greek Yogurt

- -

The Protein-Packed Probiotic Powerhouse

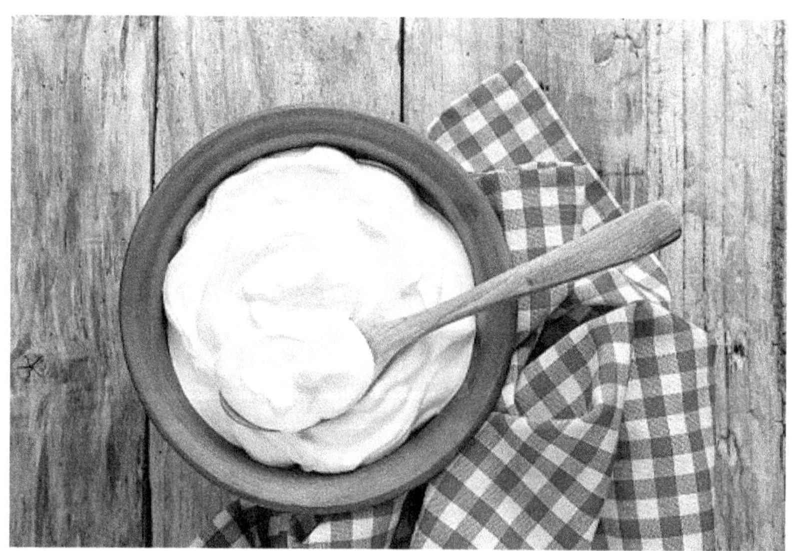

Greek yogurt, with its rich, creamy texture and tangy flavor, is a standout in the world of dairy products. Renowned for its high protein content, calcium, and probiotics, Greek yogurt is not only delicious but also incredibly nutritious. This chapter will explore the numerous health benefits of Greek yogurt, delve into its specific contributions to overall well-being, and provide practical tips and recipes to help you incorporate this versatile food into your daily diet.

The Nutritional Profile of Greek Yogurt

Greek yogurt is nutrient-rich; providing a variety of essential vitamins, minerals, and macronutrients. A 150-gram serving of plain, nonfat Greek yogurt contains:

- Calories: 100

- Protein: 10 grams

- Fat: 0 grams

- Carbohydrates: 6 grams

- Calcium: 15% of the Daily Value (DV)

- Vitamin B12: 20% of the DV

- Potassium: 6% of the DV

- Probiotics: Varies depending on the brand, but typically

contains multiple strains of beneficial bacteria.

Greek Yogurt is good for the Gut

One of the primary benefits of Greek yogurt is its ability to support and enhance gut health. Here's how it works:

Probiotics and Gut Health

Greek yogurt is rich in probiotics, which are live bacteria that provide numerous health benefits, particularly for the digestive system. These beneficial bacteria help balance the gut microbiome, improving digestion and nutrient absorption. Regular consumption of Greek yogurt can help reduce symptoms of digestive discomfort, such as bloating and constipation, and promote overall gut health.

Improving Digestive Function

The probiotics in Greek yogurt support the growth of healthy bacteria in the gut, which is crucial for maintaining a balanced digestive system. A healthy gut microbiome can enhance immune function, reduce inflammation, and even improve mental health by producing neurotransmitters like serotonin.

Greek Yogurt helps with Muscle Recovery

Greek yogurt is a favorite among fitness enthusiasts due to its high protein content, which plays a crucial role in muscle repair and recovery. Here's how it supports your fitness goals:

High Protein Content

Protein is essential for muscle repair and growth, especially after intense exercise. Greek yogurt provides a substantial amount of protein in each serving, making it an ideal post-workout snack. Consuming protein-rich foods like Greek yogurt after exercise helps repair muscle fibers, reduce muscle soreness, and promote muscle synthesis.

Amino Acids for Recovery

Greek yogurt contains all nine essential amino acids, which are the building blocks of protein. These amino acids are vital for repairing damaged muscle tissues and supporting new muscle growth. Including Greek yogurt in your diet ensures you get a complete protein source that aids in muscle recovery and overall fitness.

Promote Bone Health with Greek Yogurt

Greek yogurt is an excellent source of calcium, a mineral that is crucial for maintaining strong and healthy bones. Here's how it supports bone health:

Calcium for Strong Bones

Calcium is essential for the development and maintenance of strong bones and teeth. Adequate calcium intake helps prevent osteoporosis, a condition characterized by weak and brittle bones. Greek yogurt provides a significant amount of calcium per serving, helping you meet your daily calcium needs and supporting bone density.

Vitamin D and Bone Health

Many brands of Greek yogurt are fortified with vitamin D, which enhances calcium absorption and bone mineralization. Vitamin D works synergistically with calcium to maintain bone health, making Greek yogurt a comprehensive food for supporting your skeletal system.

Delicious Ways to Enjoy Greek Yogurt

Incorporating Greek yogurt into your diet can be both easy and delicious. Here are some creative ways to enjoy this nutrient-rich food:

Greek Yogurt with Fruit and Granola

Greek yogurt pairs perfectly with fruit and granola for a nutritious and satisfying breakfast or snack. Here's a simple recipe:

Ingredients:

- 1 cup of plain Greek yogurt

- 1/2 cup of fresh berries (strawberries, blueberries, or raspberries)

- 1/4 cup of granola

- 1 tablespoon of honey (optional)

Instructions:

1. Spoon the Greek yogurt into a bowl.

2. Top with fresh berries and granola.

3. Drizzle with honey if desired.

4. Enjoy immediately.

Greek Yogurt Smoothies

Using Greek yogurt as a base for smoothies adds creaminess and a protein boost. Here's a simple smoothie recipe:

Ingredients:

- 1 cup of Greek yogurt

- 1 banana

- 1/2 cup of frozen berries

- 1/2 cup of spinach leaves

- 1 cup of almond milk or any milk of your choice

- 1 tablespoon of honey or maple syrup (optional)

Instructions:

1. Place all ingredients in a blender.

2. Blend until smooth.

3. Pour into a glass and enjoy immediately.

Greek Yogurt Salad Dressing

Greek yogurt can be used as a base for creamy salad dressings. Here's a simple recipe:

Ingredients:

- 1/2 cup of Greek yogurt

- 2 tablespoons of olive oil

- 1 tablespoon of lemon juice

- 1 clove of garlic, minced

- 1 teaspoon of Dijon mustard

- Salt and pepper to taste

Instructions:

1. In a small bowl, whisk together the Greek yogurt, olive oil, lemon juice, minced garlic, and Dijon mustard.

2. Season with salt and pepper to taste.

3. Use as a dressing for your favorite salads.

Greek Yogurt Recipes to Try

Here are a few more delicious recipes to help you incorporate Greek yogurt into your diet:

Greek Yogurt Parfait

Ingredients:

- 1 cup of Greek yogurt

- 1/2 cup of mixed berries

- 1/4 cup of granola

- 1 tablespoon of honey (optional)

- Mint leaves for garnish (optional)

Instructions:

1. In a glass or bowl, layer half of the Greek yogurt.

2. Add half of the mixed berries and granola.

3. Repeat the layers with the remaining Greek yogurt, berries, and granola.

4. Drizzle with honey if desired.

5. Garnish with mint leaves before serving.

6. Enjoy immediately.

Greek Yogurt Dip

Ingredients:

- 1 cup of Greek yogurt

- 1 tablespoon of olive oil

- 1 tablespoon of lemon juice

- 1 clove of garlic, minced

- 1 tablespoon of fresh dill, chopped

- Salt and pepper to taste

- Fresh vegetables for dipping (carrots, cucumbers, bell peppers, etc.)

Instructions:

1. In a bowl, combine the Greek yogurt, olive oil, lemon juice, minced garlic, and chopped dill.

2. Season with salt and pepper to taste.

3. Mix well to combine.

4. Serve with fresh vegetables for dipping.

Greek Yogurt Pancakes

Ingredients:

- 1 cup of Greek yogurt

- 1 egg

- 1/2 cup of whole wheat flour

- 1 teaspoon of baking powder

- 1/2 teaspoon of baking soda

- 1 tablespoon of honey or maple syrup

- 1 teaspoon of vanilla extract

Instructions:

1. In a bowl, whisk together the Greek yogurt and egg until well combined.

2. Add the whole wheat flour, baking powder, baking soda, honey or maple syrup, and vanilla extract.

3. Stir until just combined (the batter will be thick).

4. Heat a non-stick skillet or griddle over medium heat.

5. Pour 1/4 cup of batter onto the skillet for each pancake.

6. Cook until bubbles form on the surface, then flip and cook until golden brown.

7. Serve warm with your favorite toppings.

Greek yogurt is a protein-packed, calcium-rich food that supports gut health, aids in muscle recovery, and promotes bone health. By incorporating Greek yogurt into your diet through the practical tips and delicious recipes provided, you can enjoy the many advantages of this versatile dairy product. The health benefits of Greek yogurt can transform your diet one creamy bite at a time.

Sharing the Journey to Better Health

Now you have everything you need to transform your health with nature's best nutrient-rich foods, it's time to pass on your newfound knowledge and show other readers where they can find the same help.

Scan to leave review

Please share with other health enthusiasts where they can find the information they're looking for, and pass their passion forward. The journey to better health is kept alive when we pass on our knowledge – and you're helping to do just that. Thank you for your help.

Afterword

Final Thoughts

Throughout this book, we have explored the many benefits of ten powerful superfoods that can significantly enhance your health and well-being, hence affording you a better quality of life, if applied. These nutrient-rich foods—kale, blueberries, salmon, spinach, quinoa, avocado, chia seeds, broccoli, sweet potatoes, and Greek yogurt—are not only rich in essential vitamins and minerals but also packed with antioxidants, healthy fats, and fiber that support various aspects of your health.

By incorporating these superfoods into your diet, you can take proactive steps towards boosting your immune system, improving heart health, enhancing cognitive function, and maintaining overall vitality. The goal is not just to eat healthily but to savor the delicious and nutritious flavors that these foods bring to your table.

I hope that this book has inspired you to experiment with other recipes besides those included here and find creative ways to add these superfoods to your meals. From vibrant salads and hearty soups to refreshing smoothies and wholesome snacks, there are endless possibilities to enjoy the benefits of these nutritional powerhouses.

A quick side note; I had a short report made on burning fat that highlights 16 key factors I think can help keep fat gain to a minimum by understanding how to get your body to burn more fat.
Scan the QR-code to download the free report.

As you continue your journey towards better health, remember to keep these superfoods at the top of your grocery list. With a kitchen stocked with these ingredients, you will be well-equipped to nourish your body and enjoy eating well.

Thank you for joining me on this journey. Here's to a healthier, happier you—filled with the energy and vitality that comes from embracing the power of superfoods. To your health and well-being!

About the Author

Conard Howe is an inspiring figure from Harlem, New York, a husband, and father of 5 children, known for his passion for music and technology he utilizes both to create unique works in his space. He has held various influential roles, including management positions in different sectors of the music and broadcast industry, and is now a co-owner of Genius Mindz LLC | Content Promo-Ai .com.

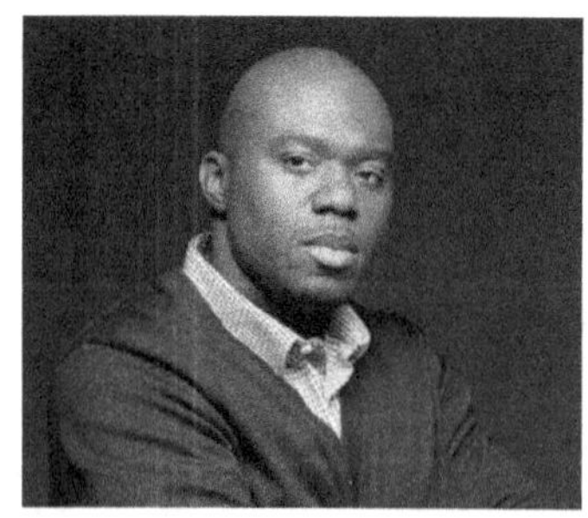

As a small business consultant, his work focuses on creating strategies to keep customers coming back and building strong relationships for clients with their current and potential customers, something he calls "Backend Automation Retention Strategies" or B.A.R.S. He shares the lessons he has learned along the way in his writings, aiming to help others overcome their challenges and reach their full potential.

Joining Conard on his journey means to set out on a path of transformation and discovery. He aims to motivate his readers to overcome obstacles and unlock their boundless potential. With his unique blend of technical skill and creative thinking, he offers insights that encourage you to live the life you've always wanted.

Conard's story is not just remarkable—it's a guide to living a life filled with innovation, growth, and success.

Also by

***

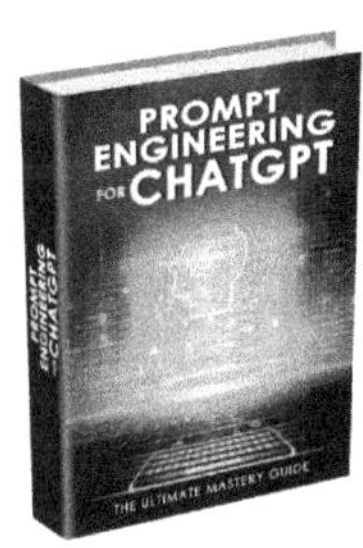

Now on Amazon

Prompt Engineering for ChatGPT. This comprehensive guide, details innovative prompting strategies and techniques that enhance ChatGPT's responsiveness, so the output you get is more closely related to what you want. This allows anyone to turn ChatGPT into an indispensable tool for personal and/or business use.

scan to leave your review

***

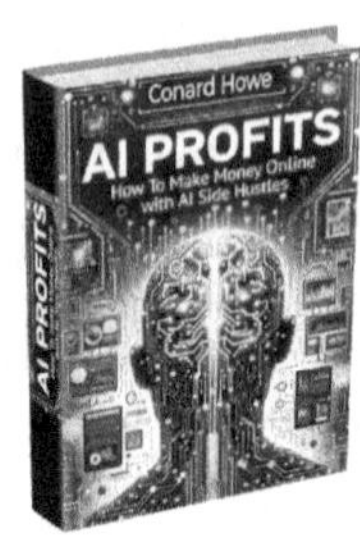

Now on Amazon

AI Profits. The AI boom of 2022 created a new digital landscape, a playground of profitability; arm yourself with the knowledge of how to navigate AI driven platforms, use AI tools and create profitable AI side hustles to create passive online income; lots of it. "Get Yours!" –CNBC

scan to leave your review

***

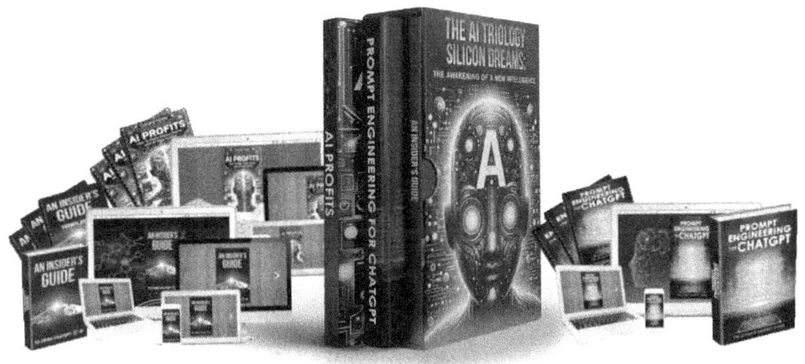

The *Silicon Dreams* box set bundle merges my three essential guide books on ChatGPT:

1. An Insider's Guide to Using ChatGPT A.I.

2. Prompt Engineering for ChatGPT

3. AI Profits

I've bundled additional resources to compliment the boxset, to ensure you get the most out of every interaction.

Each volume offers practical, actionable insights to boost creativity, increase business productivity, improve on academic research, and opens the door to AI-centric income opportunities.

Want to unlock all the potential AI has to offer and the many ways to benefit from your newfound understanding of it? This will help!

scan to leave your review

***

**THE
END**